Yesid Ramírez Moya
Clara Lida Beltrán Beltrán

Safe practices in low complexity home care

Yesid Ramírez Moya
Clara Lida Beltrán Beltrán

Safe practices in low complexity home care

How to improve the safety of home care, based on the investigation of its risk factors

ScienciaScripts

Imprint

Any brand names and product names mentioned in this book are subject to trademark, brand or patent protection and are trademarks or registered trademarks of their respective holders. The use of brand names, product names, common names, trade names, product descriptions etc. even without a particular marking in this work is in no way to be construed to mean that such names may be regarded as unrestricted in respect of trademark and brand protection legislation and could thus be used by anyone.

Cover image: www.ingimage.com

This book is a translation from the original published under ISBN 978-3-659-00337-0.

Publisher:
Sciencia Scripts
is a trademark of
Dodo Books Indian Ocean Ltd. and OmniScriptum S.R.L publishing group

120 High Road, East Finchley, London, N2 9ED, United Kingdom
Str. Armeneasca 28/1, office 1, Chisinau MD-2012, Republic of Moldova, Europe
Printed at: see last page
ISBN: 978-620-5-61079-4

Contents

Dedication

Writing this work is the product of my concern and passion for patient safety, but this initiative takes more strength when I become a support for the care of my father, to whom I dedicate this work, because with his illness he taught me the need to take care of the patient and the family at home.

Yesid Ram^ez Moya

I dedicate this work to each and every patient who requires home care and for whom we, as health professionals, must give the best of our knowledge based on life experience.

Clara Lida Beltran

Acknowledgements

To Virrey SoKs IPS and its health team, who very kindly opened the doors of the institution and their knowledge to carry out this study.

To the Fundacion Universitaria Juan N. Corpas and the Master of Public Health, who motivated us and gave us the opportunity to express our knowledge in this research work.

To Dr. Alvaro Quintero, who with his knowledge and teachings inspired us to develop this work in a comprehensive manner.

To the patients and relatives of the home care programme, who gave us their experiences in a disinterested and very collaborative way for a better understanding of this model of care.

To our families who encouraged us not to give up trying to make this dream a reality.

Glossary

• Patient safety: It is defined as the "set of structural elements, processes, instruments and methodologies based on scientifically proven evidence that seek to minimise the risk of suffering an adverse event in the health care process or to mitigate its consequences. It involves the ongoing assessment of the risks associated with health care in order to design and implement the necessary safety barriers" (1).

• Health care: "Services received by individuals or populations to promote, maintain, monitor or restore health" (2).

• Indication of unsafe care: "An event or circumstance that may alert to an increased risk of an incident or adverse event occurring" (2).

• Adverse event: "The result of health care that unintentionally resulted in harm. Adverse events can be preventable and non-preventable" (2).

• Preventable adverse event: "An unintended, undesirable, unintended outcome that could have been avoided by adherence to the standards of care available at the time" (2).

• Unpreventable adverse event: "Unintended, undesirable, unintended outcome that occurs despite compliance with standards of care" (2).

• Incident: "It is an event or circumstance that occurs in a patient's medical care that does not cause harm, but whose occurrence incorporates failures in the care processes" (2).

• Home care: Modality of out-of-hospital health service provision that seeks to provide a solution to health problems in the home or residence, with the support of health professionals, technicians or auxiliaries and the participation of the family.

• Palliative care: Appropriate care for the patient with a chronic, terminal, degenerative and irreversible pathology where the control of pain and other symptoms requires, in addition to medical, social and spiritual support, psychological and family support during illness and bereavement. The aim is to achieve the best possible quality of life for the patient and family. It regards dying as a normal process.

- Hospitalisation service: "It is the service that provides health care to patients who, due to their health condition, require a hospital stay of more than 24 hours for follow-up or for the performance of procedures, in the case of home care it applies to low complexity services; it will be provided with controlled criteria, with the support of health professionals, technicians or assistants and the participation of the family or a caregiver" (6).

Summary

Home-based services provide care for patients who, because of their medical condition, remain with spermatological care at home. Being the user's residence a place not made for health care, it offers additional risks to those of a hospital environment, therefore, they require specific guidelines and orientations for their implementation. Based on the analysis of knowledge and experiences of events and incidents in home care, we propose good and safe practices for this model of care, favouring coordinated work among its actors, with emphasis on risk management by providers, caregivers and patients in low complexity care. This descriptive observational study includes a bibliographic search of information related to safe practices in home care; the analysis of adverse events in a low complexity home care institution that allows to characterize the main events identified; semi-structured surveys to professionals, patients, caregivers and Kderes of the system, aimed at collecting knowledge and experiences on guidelines and safe practices implemented. The results showed that in the articles found, no proposals for safe practices were identified; the main adverse events in home care were characterised; the lack of specific safe practices for professionals, patients and carers on event prevention and risk management in this model of care was noted. It was therefore concluded that it is essential to propose four packages of safe practices that aim to strengthen safety in home care, involving actors of the system, with emphasis on providers, and recommendations on the importance of the caregiver and self-care of the patient and family.

Keywords: patient safety, home care, adverse events, good safety practices.

Introduction

Through home services, care is provided to patients whose pathological condition and disability limit their attendance at the service centres. Likewise, care processes that do not involve hospitalisation can be carried out at home by a trained interdisciplinary team, offering care in the patient's home environment, involving their family and carers in this process.

The home environment generates additional risk factors such as nutrition, hygiene, self-care, ambulation and in 30% of the cases there are dysfunctional families that increase the unsafe conditions for the patient care process.

Safe practices are the path that patient safety has followed in other care settings and is the benchmark we have in home care today, but according to the knowledge gained and experiences known, it is necessary to adjust them specifically to a home care setting.

The development of this work coincided with one of the greatest tests in terms of public health that the world has undergone in the last decade, which led to the search for health care alternatives that would generate care with less risk of contagion, that would allow continuity of care and that found in home care a transitory solution for such acute care and, in passing, ensure continuity of care for the chronic pathologies that have increased in the last 45 years.

Patient safety in home care as a public health event is the responsibility of the State and the actors in the health system. In order to make an integrated proposal that manages the risks inherent to this care, it is necessary to characterise the population that is the object of the proposal, as well as to identify the risks involved in this type of care.

- The State, represented by the Ministry of Health and Social Protection, as the governing body, should contemplate specific guidelines to address the problem of safety in home-based care in Colombia, since the regulations in force so far assume it as an extension of hospital services or as a variety of outpatient care.
- The territorial bodies as managers of the MAITE (7) integrated territorial care model must be the guarantors of care for the population of the different territories and under their tutelage is the functioning of the care networks as the basis for the provision of health services for all people; they must give a differential character and strict monitoring to this modality of care.
- At another level we have the administrators and providers who are responsible

for risk management and the delivery of the different models of care, respectively, and in the hands of these organisations lies the operationalisation of a risk prevention model in home-based care.

• Fourth and not least are the patients and their families who suffer, ultimately, the impact of adverse events occurring during the provision of the service, to the detriment of their own lives and family stability.

In order to develop an integrative proposal for safe practices in low complexity home care, it was necessary to develop a methodology that allowed us to start from existing knowledge at international and national level, and then explore how this service has been provided in our Colombia, through the review of the performance of safety in care in a patient safety programme in a low complexity home health institution; to make a comprehensive analysis it was necessary to make a diagnosis that would inform about the occurrence of events in home care, collecting the experiences of professionals, patients and caregivers, who provided valuable information, which allowed greater knowledge of the conditions of home care.

Each group of patients requires a differential approach according to their pathology and the programme in which they have been classified, which involves a planning process associated with specific protocols based on clinical practice guidelines, exhaustive follow-up and correct decision making. This care requires the work of an interdisciplinary team, which through coordinated activity and with the help of biomedical technology, guarantees the safe provision of services at home.

Problem statement

The provision of health services seeks in home care alternatives with better opportunity, at lower costs, increasing the coverage of health services, with a more humanised care, in the patient's familiar environment, with the support of the family.

But it should be taken into account that this care will be provided in a home environment, which is adapted for housing and not for providing medical care, making the provision of health care more risky, facilitating the occurrence of events that can range from an indication of unsafe care, to the occurrence of adverse events that could lead to the death of the patient, being these events mostly preventable, through the implementation of some measures, which are called good practices of safety in care.

The prevalence of these adverse events identified in Colombia in a related study in a home care programme in Bogota (2014-2015) (3) was 1.0% and a review in the Revista de salud publica CES. Sanchez M, Fuentes G. Gestion cHnica de programas de cuidado domiciliario (4) report some adverse events typical of home care and some of their causes, proposing some interventions such as training, education and training of the health professional and the caregiver, in relation to the management of the programme, with a focus on risk and taking into account care strategies derived from chronicity and longevity, suggesting a cost-effective and safe option.

In relation to the intervention of adverse events in the home care model, Law 100 in 1993 (5) lacks specific regulations, an aspect which has obliged health institutions and some local authorities to create and organise their own home care models and programmes based on programmes created in other countries, adopting them to the national context, without effective risk control; perhaps aiming more at greater coverage, better opportunity, better comfort, but without defining minimum levels of safety in the care process. While little risk control is identified at the home level, there is work on safe care at the hospital and outpatient level, based on the best available evidence, but no research is identified at the home level that proposes a better coordination of the actors in the system in order to intervene in risks related to the characteristics of home care, taking into account the local conditions, human talent, as well as the processes and procedures that involve risks specific to the home.

In addition to the failures related to health care, there are contributory factors related to the absence of a national policy that includes coordination between the state, control bodies, administrators, providers and users in order to reduce the failures that arise from the lack of integration of the different actors in the system.

Home care is assumed to be a derivation of outpatient or inpatient care, ignoring the risks inherent in home care and the involvement of caregivers who are not sufficiently trained and whose processes are different from those provided in inpatient care or within health facilities in outpatient care.

The single system of habilitation shows very basic requirements for the home setting and whose requirements are limited to minimum requirements for the provider (6) and requirements for the administrator, related to timeliness of care and the provision of support services that the user needs; all of them assumed as part of outpatient care, without taking into account the risks inherent to home care.

In addition to the care risks identified in home care, there is a gap related to identifying and responding to the needs and expectations of patients and carers, which, if they can be studied and intervened, could make this service more humanised and safer.

With the results of the present research, it was proposed to create an integrative tool that provides the different actors of the system with safe practices and procedures, improving the coordination of their interventions, impacting the quality of care at home, minimising risks for patients and their families.

The proposed integration proposal focused on the identification and prioritisation of risks and needs in the home environment, starting from the limitations and specifications of the home environment.

From what was identified as a result of the research it was possible to establish that health teams should be prepared for home management; with provider institutions and training centres aware of this responsibility, promoting qualified human talent and the training of caregivers, trained to meet the requirements of home care.

Among the limitations of this project were: The scarce definition of a public policy for the intervention of risks related to home care, as well as the deficient information related to the triggers of adverse events and unsafe care at home, as well as the lack of information received by patients and caregivers regarding the identification of adverse events and incidents in this type of care.

If this project had not been carried out, it would have limited the generation of expected guidelines for the effective management of home care, which would favour adequate coordination between the actors in the system, in the development of safe practices and procedures between institutions, health professionals, patients and caregivers, in order to improve safety and quality in the field of home care in Colombia.

4.1 General objective

To formulate an integrated proposal for safe home care with effective management guidelines, through adequate coordination between the actors in the system, for the development of safe practices and procedures by institutions, health professionals, patients and caregivers, for the benefit of the safety and quality of home care in Colombia.

4.2 Specific objectives:

1.   Identify documentary evidence related to safe home care practices, in the last 5 years (2016 to 2020), in national and international databases.
2.   To identify and characterise adverse events reported in a low complexity home care IPS, during a period of 3 years (2018 to 2020), and their main causes.

3.   To characterise the experience of home care and its main risks from the knowledge of patients, carers and treating professionals.
4.   To evaluate the applicability, scope and results of the implementation of existing guidelines for the prevention of adverse events and unsafe care in a low complexity home care service, from the perspective of the health system's thematic referents.

Patient safety and its relation to primary health care (PHC)

Primary health care is the patient's gateway to the health system, which makes it necessary to have safe practices to prevent the occurrence of events or incidents in their care.

The services provided in primary health care include: disease prevention, health promotion, education in healthy lifestyles, diagnosis and treatment phases, as well as palliative care.

Through the patient safety programme, we intervene in the risks that arise during the care process. We must manage situations inherent to lack of opportunity for care, geographic and cultural barriers, errors in diagnosis or treatment, those related to technological or infrastructure aspects, lack of some services not covered by the benefit plan and other situations that put the patient's integrity at risk.

APEAS study: (8)

A study conducted in Spain on patient safety in primary health care, Ministry of Health and Consumer Affairs, Madrid Spain 2008, reveals that, for primary health care services, a prevalence of 11.2 adverse events per 100 visits is identified, 70% of which are avoidable and mostly related to medication and care in care (70%), to a lesser extent communication-related events (24%) and management-related events (8.9%). As shown in table 1.

Table 1. Adverse events in Apeas study

CONCEPT		RESULT	
Prevalence rate of adverse events		11.2 Adverse Events per 1000 visits	
Avoidable events			
Related to medication and care			
Related to communication		24.6	
Management-related8	.9% Management-related8	.9% Management-related8	.9%
Management-related8	.9% Management-related8	.9% Management-related8	.9%
	Management-related		

Note: APEAS Project.

AMBEAS study (9)

A study defined for the analysis of incidence, prevalence and origin of adverse events in patients attending ambulatory care services, carried out in Brazil, Colombia, Mexico and Peru, during the years 2010-2012, shows that among the risk factors related to adverse events generated in ambulatory care, those related to poor information to the user stand out in 22.9%; incomplete clinical records in 14.4%, little time dedicated to the patient by the professional in 20.5%, factors inherent to the patient in 22.8%, problems related to doctor-patient communication in 7.2%, lack of adherence to guidelines in 7.2% and some failures of the professional related to fatigue and distractions in 3.6%, as shown in table 2.

Table 2. Risks in care identified in the Ambeas study

RISKS IDENTIFIED	PERCENTAGE OF OCCURRENCE	
Insufficient knowledge	22.9%	
Incomplete physical examination		14.4%

Lack of time		20.5%
Uncooperative patient		10.8%
Patient complexity	12%	
Lack of guidelines		7.2%
Lack of patient understanding. Professional		7.2%
Distractions/professional fatigue		3.6%

Note: AMBEAS Project.

Today Colombia has a National Patient Safety Policy (10) and a Technical Guide of Good Safety Practices (11), designed on the basis of evidence-based medicine or expert recommendations, which minimise risk and promote safe care, applicable to inpatient and outpatient settings, with no difference for the home setting.

Chapter 2

Theoretical framework

Patient safety changes according to the context: Most of the learning done so far has its origins in the analysis and learning that has been done in the hospital setting and from alif adaptations have been made to the outpatient setting; but for the home setting other analyses and learning are necessary, taking into account the risks of the home, the poor training of caregivers, the lack of technological support, the lack of timely follow-up and treatment to which the patient can sometimes be exposed in the home setting, as shown in table 3.

Table 3. Comparison of controls for major adverse events in different care settings.

EVENT O INCIDENT	ENVIRONMENT	OUTPATIENT SETTING	HOME ENVIRONMENT
PRESCRIPTION **errors**	More opportunity for monitoring between nursing and pharmacy staff.	Control depends on patient o caregiver autonomy	Control depends on patient autonomy o caregiver
ERRORS OF medicines administration	More can be avoided with trained personnel and appropriate technology.	Depends on autonomy of patient o caregiver	Depends on autonomy of patient o caregiver
FALLS	MasBarreras by special infrastructure personalalexclusive trained	Infrastructure y adequate staffing at y the time of care y increased risk at y home	Infrastructure is a latent risk, so coto the staff caring for the patient at home.
COMMUNICATION **failures**	They can be mitigated with the participation of several health professionals who monitor on an ongoing basis	It is only mitigated at the time of consultation.	Only partially handled at the time of the visit by health personnel.
PHLEBITIS	Rapidly identified y monitored by health personnel	Only identified at the time of the visit	Only identified if there is support from health personnel.
vascular catheter infection	More health professional shift monitors	Susceptible to control only in the consultation o control in the IPS	Control only at the time of the home visit.
CLERICAL ERRORS	Less frequent by permanent monitoring by the health team	Moderately manageable when visiting the health institution	More difficult to resolve from the patient's home y by the caregiver
ERRORS RELATED TO LABORATORY SAMPLES	More likely to be remedied during the shift o hospitalisation	More delayed resolution until the next consultation.	More delayed its resolution until the home visit.

Among the main adverse events prioritised by different international agencies mainly for inpatient and outpatient care settings, 16 events have been identified whose occurrence varies in the different settings, some of them being present in the home setting with some very particular risk factors. Within this prioritisation are those listed in table 4.

Table 4. Prioritisation of adverse events by international agencies

Agency for healthcare Research and Quality (2013)	National Quality Forum (2010)	Joint Commission (2014)	QMS Patient Safety Solutions (2014)
Hand hygiene	Hand hygiene	Hand hygiene	Hand hygiene
Drug reconciliation	High-risk medicines	Reconciliation Medicamentosa	Medication reconciliation
High-risk medicines Safe surgery	Safe surgery	Safe surgery	High-risk medicines
Safe surgery	Catheter-associated bacteraemia	Catheter-associated bacteraemia	Safe surgery
Catheter bacteraemia	Bladder catheter infection	Urinary catheter infection	Transition of care

Bladder catheter-related infection	Surgical infection	Surgical infection	Medicinal products with the name y look a like, sound a like (Look a like, sound a like)
Ventilator-associated pneumomia	Ventilator-associated pneumonia	Id.	
Medical devices	Medical devices	Communication	
Transition of care	Informed consent		
Pressure ulcers	Transition of care		
Falls	Antimicrobial resistance		
Patient or caregiver responsibility			
	Pressure ulcers		
	Falls -Thrombosis Venous		

Note. Patient safety strategy of the national health system. Period 2015-2020

To control these identified adverse events, safe practices and procedures are in place, which are interventions aimed at preventing or mitigating unnecessary harm associated with health care and improving safety in patient care (11).

They are the product of learning from the research, analysis and improvement of risks identified and managed in different health institutions around the world.

Patient safety can be improved by reducing the likelihood of adverse events by eliminating the activity that causes them, if possible, by avoiding human error in the performance of the activity or by controlling system failures; by acting in advance of the occurrence of harm or, if events have already occurred, by intervening in a timely manner to mitigate their effects.

Good patient safety practices have been widely studied and put into practice in hospital care settings, at the primary care level they have been strengthened, with the identification of unsafe care and adverse events, and in the home setting it is necessary to strengthen them in order to generate comprehensive care models that have a preventive focus on the patient, their family and carers, who, being autonomous in decision-making and actions, generate greater exposure to risks, unsafe care and adverse events; Among these are adverse drug reactions, infections, falls, ulcers, thrombotic processes, etc.

In the intervention of these adverse events, an analysis of the patient's environment must be carried out in a systematic manner, generating preventive, supervised care models, with regulatory standards and with the scope of the governing body (Ministry of Health and Social Protection); control body (Supersalud and territorial entities); administrators (entities administering benefit plans), providers (institutions providing services) and users.

In home-based care, the main errors are due to omission, lack of access to timely care and lack of supervision, additionally, depending on the event, repetitive failures can be considered as requiring intervention.

Home care demands greater attention from the treating health professional, as well as nursing and family/caregiver care. Every patient in home care requires greater emphasis on self-care measures, as well as education of the caregiver and strict follow-up by the health care team. Each patient should be assessed in an individual context of risk estimation, diagnosis, prognosis and personalised management plan (12).

Within the context of palliative care, this type of care generally involves education in routine care, attention to urgent, minor or common health problems, mental health care, psychosocial services, health promotion and disease prevention, nutritional counselling and end-of-life care. All of these are aimed at avoiding or mitigating major injuries or additional damage to the patient (13).

In the home setting, patients and caregivers play a key role in diagnosis, management and interventions, including at critical moments when they are the decision-makers and non-decision-makers. Professionals consider that the home setting generates greater risk because there are no health personnel to monitor the patient, who is left in the care of an untrained caregiver.

The home care model must be strengthened in the identification and management of the risks inherent to the home, guaranteeing minimum conditions for the provision of health services that allow for: prevention of infections, order and cleanliness, prevention of falls, mobilisation procedures for prostrate patients, adequate administration of medicines, use of personal protective equipment, possibility of transmission of infections between homes due to the movement of personnel, inadequate hand washing and disinfection of equipment.

It is essential to take into account in the home care model the strengthening of the competencies of family members and caregivers who assume the role, the acceptance of the environment of a patient in chronic condition, hospitalised at home or in palliative care. Likewise, the role of the home care aide is very important and should be adequately trained in the administration of medication. When the patient receives visits from professionals from different disciplines, it is seen as a fragmentation of the care model, generating greater risks due to ambiguity of concepts and practices in the treatment plan.

5.1 Legislation in Colombia on home-based care

In terms of legislation in Colombia, home-based care services are regulated and are described in table 5.

Table 5. Legislation in Colombia on home-based care

Law 1122 of 2007	Improvement in the provision of services to users.
Resolution 13431 of 1991	Hospital Ethics Committees are established and the Decalogue of Patients' Rights is adopted.
Resolution 1995 of 1999	Whereby the parameters for compliance with the rules for the management of medical records are established.
Resolution 5928 of 2016	Requirements for the recognition and payment of the caregiver service, as an exceptional service financed by the SGSSS.
Resolution 6406 of 2016	Modifies health benefit plan **Article 26**: Home care as an alternative to hospital care **Artfeuio 68**: Palliative Care in Home Care **Article 82**: Care for the recovery of health: benefit plan covers any outpatient, inpatient or home care, with focus on RIAS- MIAS and PAIS
Resolution 839 of 2017	Article 1: Handling, custody, retention time, preservation and final disposition of medical records,
Resolution 3100 of 2019	Establishes the modalities of service provision and infrastructure criteria for home-based care.
Judgment T-065/18	Right to health: Double connotation as a fundamental right and at the same time a public service. Fundamental Right to Health: Special Constitutional Protection Provision of nursing and home care: To be guaranteed by the EPSs from the resources they receive.

Chapter 3

Methodology

A descriptive observational study whose methodology was implemented for each of the objectives as follows:

1. Identify documentary evidence related to safe home care practices in the last 5 years (2016 to 2020) in national and international databases.

1.1 Data collection

A documentary review was carried out using a search of databases from the last 5 years (2015-2020), worldwide (Pubmed), Latin American (Redalyc) and national academic databases (Repositories of universities that have related studies. Redcol).

1.2 Information analysis

A search was carried out using indicated search engines using keywords in English and Spanish: adverse events, home care, risks in care, home care, health care service at home,

1.3 Measurement level

Existence of publications on safe practices in low complexity home care; product of the identification of adverse events and their causes.

2   To identify and characterise adverse events reported, in a low complexity home care IPS, during a period of 3 years (2018 to 2020) and their main causes.

2.1 Data collection

Prior to the documentary review of the selected low complexity home care IPS, we had the approval of the research ethics committee, guaranteeing confidentiality and the handling of information such as: home care protocol, adverse events report (2018 to 2020), risk classification matrix; access to patient database and the home adverse events report database.

2.2 Information analysis

Information reported on adverse events in chronic, critical non-ventilator care, home hospitalisation and palliative care was taken into account.

Based on the prioritisation of adverse events and with the help of the problem-based approach methodology presented by the Ministry of Health and Social Protection of Colombia in 2016, Figure 1, the London protocol analysis was applied to the main adverse events identified.

The result of these analyses of active failures, contributory factors and latent failures, which have been identified around the prioritised adverse events in home care, is presented in such a way that a proposal for "safe practices" for the intervention of the prioritised adverse events is constructed on the basis of this causal analysis.

Figure 1. Model of the problem-based approach suggested by the Ministry of Health and Social Protection

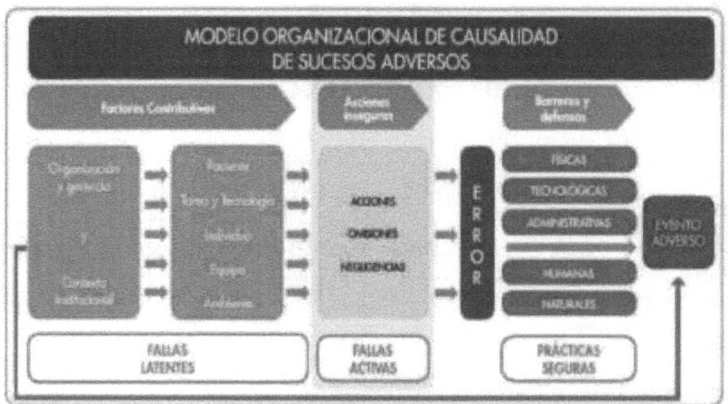

Note: LONDON PROTOCOL, Sally Taylor-Adams and Charles Vincent (Clinical Safety Research Unit, Imperial College London, UK).

2.3 Measurement level

Indicators such as overall rate of adverse events and type of event, causes of adverse events reported and improvement actions implemented, other variables such as age, gender, type of care and associated diagnosis were evaluated.

3 To characterise the experience of home care and its main risks from the knowledge of patients, carers and treating professionals.

3.1 Data collection

The experience of patients in the programme and caregivers was characterised through directed surveys; with the professionals, surveys were conducted on the perception of risks in the patient's environment, associated human factors, materials and existing controls. These surveys were carried out after filling out an informed consent form, explaining to the participants the objectives of the research, the procedure to be carried out, possible risks and benefits, availability to respond to concerns, freedom to participate or not in the research, protection of confidentiality and of the information and the strict and specific use of the same.

A survey was programmed to six professionals of the home care programme, but given the importance of the role of the occupational therapist in the management and rehabilitation process of the home patient, this professional was included as a seventh survey to be carried out, so that a group of seven professionals of the home care service were surveyed.

One social worker; two doctors; two nursing assistants; one nurse; one occupational therapist, applying 15 questions related to the identification of good safety practices, technical guidelines of the home-based programme, service risks, measurement of the impact of the practice, detection of adverse events related to the provision of the service.

3.2 Analysis of the information

By means of the perception of risks during the provision of the service and of existing preventive actions, the aspects of this care process became known.

3.3 Measurement level

The surveys assessed the perceived risks to the service's activities, as well as the existence of controls and possible causes of these risks.

4.   The applicability, scope and results of the implementation of existing guidelines for the prevention of adverse events and unsafe care in a low complexity home care service were evaluated from the perspective of the health system's thematic referents.

4.1 Information gathering: Surveys were used to clarify issues related to existing guidelines on safety in home care, risk control activities in low complexity home care.

4.2 A survey was carried out with five health system referents to identify safety guidelines in home care: a quality referent from the Ministry of Health and Social Protection, a referent from a health secretariat, a director of a company providing home health services, a manager of a home services company, and a referent from the safety programme of the service provider.

4.3 Analysis of the information

Through surveys of health system stakeholders, we sought to validate information related to existing controls to prevent adverse events and incidents in home-based care.

4.4 Measurement level

Through the surveys of these referents, the existing measures and their effectiveness in intervening the main risks of home-based care, safety barriers implemented (safe practices), level of implementation and possible impact were validated.

Types of study variables:

Dependent variables: The main adverse events identified in low complexity home care were reviewed.

Independent variables: Causes related to these adverse events were identified, such as age, gender, associated diseases, existence or non-existence of information by the health team to patients and carers, mainly.

Chapter 4

Results

For the integrative proposal for safe practices in low complexity home care, an approach by each of the stakeholders was planted as shown in Table 6.

Table 6. Stakeholders in the system and proposal

Stakeholder in the system	Agent Proposals
Governing body	Guidelines for the strengthening of the policy of Ministry of Health home-based care services y of the Ministry of Health. Patient safety policy in Colombia
Technical advice: Surveillance and control	Minimum requirements for the provision of home care . Health Secretariats' guidelines for a comprehensive security programme for the Departmental y Distntales. patient in home care providers.
Administrators	Criteria for the procurement y provision of home care services
Providers	Ips Practice y safe home care procedures for providers y users. including caregivers
Users	Recommendations for a caregiver profile, Patients. family y carers recommendations to be taken into account by patients. family y carers in the Home.

In order to operationalise the integration proposal, it was proposed to gradually develop a

Action plan at the following levels of intervention, asf:

a) At the national level

• Include home-based care as an integral and indispensable element of outpatient care.

• Include good practice in home care in the national patient safety policy and in the Good Safety Practice Manual.

• Include in the existing minimum qualification requirements for home-based care.

• Reorganise the capitation payment unit (UPC) in order to finance home-based care.

- Include the technical and non-technical caregiver in the benefit plan for the care of patients at home, according to the level of affectation of each user.

b) At regional level

- Advise on the application of the national standard, both to administrators and to providers and users.
- To carry out surveillance and control of compliance with the minimum qualification requirements for home care.

c) At the level of administrators

- Have a patient safety policy and programme in place that includes home care safety.
- To monitor and control the quality and safety of home-based care.
- To cover the costs necessary to ensure the safe care of users at home.
- Implement the need to comply with the inclusion of the technical and non-technical caregiver in the care processes of the programme's patients.

d) At provider level

- Have a patient safety policy and programme in place that includes home care safety.
- To monitor and control the quality and safety of home-based care, with management indicators.
- To have the necessary resources to guarantee the safe care of its users at home.
- Train home care professionals in safe practices for the service.
- Develop administrative and care processes to ensure timely, safe and effective home-based care.

- Promote the "Care for carers" programme as part of comprehensive care for users. For which a model of safe practices is proposed.
- Take into account in the care process the guidelines for safety in home care as set out in the "Cartilla de prácticas seguras en atención domiciliaria de baja complejidad", which is part of Annex A.

Within the care procedures, the provision of care must include:

1. Criteria for entering and leaving the service
2. Medical history and records: each patient should have their own medical history

opened for the programme, with a unified history available to the health team, guaranteeing confidentiality and security, with clear, legible records, without amendments and preferably at the same time as the care provided.

3. An informed consent form must be in place for the patient or caregiver to authorise care procedures after being informed of the benefits, risks, alternatives and implications of home care.

4. The patient must have an admission assessment at the time of admission to the programme, from which an individual treatment plan tailored to the morbidity should be generated.

5. Define a referencing and counter-referencing procedure

6. Generate recommendations and care by interdisciplinary health personnel, according to the scope of care received by the patient.

7. It should have a description of the care provided by the caregiver if required.

8. With regard to the provision of biomedical equipment, it must have: stethoscope, blood pressure meter, organ equipment, oximeter, glucometer, reflex hammer, thermometer, measuring tape, medical grade scales and a defined, programmed and executed maintenance plan.

9. In case of medication administration, it must comply with the specifications of the standard and have a home medication management manual (deliverables).

10. In relation to the human talent, the specifications defined for the outpatient setting apply, health professionals with degrees defined by the Ministry of Education and the due registrations for the exercise of the profession, according to profile: medical professional, nursing professional, nursing assistant. The continuous care by the health care personnel at the patient's home will be determined according to the clinical stage and the care procedures will be determined in relation to the standard of priority procedures.

11. Training should be provided to the patient, family member or caregiver, including home disinfection management, waste management, proper use and storage of medical devices and medicines.

12. For the inpatient service of the chronic patient without ventilator, the home must have an assessment of the accessibility conditions and the specifications mentioned above.

It is important to have minimum criteria for admitting a patient to a home-based care programme, such as:

1. Carry out a pre-visit to the home to define compliance with the general conditions.

2. The patient and family should follow the recommendations given by the interdisciplinary group.

3. The service must be received at the same address from the beginning of the management until the end of the services. In the event of a change of address, the administrative area of the programme must be notified in order to schedule a new inspection visit and adjust the service routes.

4. The address must have water, electricity, sewage, telephone and adequate access roads.

5. A responsible adult must be in charge of the patient and accompany him/her throughout the treatment, who reports any complications to the care team.

6. If the patient receives medication, it should be administered by medical order at set times (at 6, 8, 12 or 24 hours).

7. During the process of home care, the patient will not be able to leave the home unless he/she requires medical controls or diagnostic examinations, with prior notice to the administrative area of the programme, otherwise the patient may be excluded from the programme.

8. If the patient is hospitalised or goes to an emergency department, the person in charge must inform the administrative area of the home programme.

9. To re-enter the programme there must be a medical order from the place where you are hospitalised.

10. Once treatment is completed, the programme physician will discharge the patient and the patient will continue in outpatient services.

11. Waste management should be tight and not mixed with ordinary waste.

12. The periodicity of care is defined according to the medical order and according to morbidity.

13. The caregiver or patient must present all medical orders at the time of the visit for proper care and reformulation processes.

14. If the patient requires transfer for procedures or medical appointments, administrative arrangements must be made to ensure adequate and safe transport.

15. If the patient is hospitalised or requires emergency care, the responsible person must notify the administrative area of the programme.

16. Medical or paramedical staff visits are scheduled.

To have a specific training plan where the following topics are prioritised, which is an important practice to implement as a general guideline for users of the programme:

- Skin care
- How to prevent pressure ulcers
- How medicines should be administered safely
- Bathroom in bed
- Postural care of the caregiver

- Prevention of musculoskeletal injuries in the caregiver: tear, herniated disc, tension headache
- Infection prevention
- Effects on the caregiver's health
- Assertive communication
- Administrative formalities related to care
- Warning signs for the underlying pathology

What the profile of a home care carer should be like:

Within the assessment of caregiver competencies, we consider the following aspects, both for technical personnel who work as caregivers, as well as for non-technical and non-professional persons who must assist patients and must receive the necessary training processes for such work.

A. Caregiver technical assistant nurse in home care

Whose competency-based approach induces you to:

- Provide care and guidance to patients according to their needs and perspectives in accordance with defined guidelines and institutional policies.
- Admit the user to health services in accordance with institutional procedures.
- Control infections in patients by securing the environment with your good practices.
- Favouring the management of individual diagnosis according to guidelines and required technology.
- To assist the patient in the daily activities according to the conditions of the assigned user and with the definition of management generated by a professional

under current protocols and guidelines.

- To contribute to patient care for the maintenance and recovery of systemic functions by age group in relation to defined technical and ethical principles.
- Administration of intramuscular medication, according to medical prescription and current protocols.
- To provide comprehensive care for the individual and the family.
- Generate sociable and healthy attitudes and practices in the work environment.

B. Non-technical, non-health professional caregiver

The caregiver is a person who takes care of a patient, must be a caring and committed adult with defined physical and mental capacities, usually a close relative or a person hired by the family, the care is provided in the patient's or the family's home.

The caregiver must receive training that is closely aligned with the diseases and care required by each patient, as well as excellent communication with the health care team and serve as a bridge of communication between the health care team and the patient.

Having guidelines to promote the care of caregivers, ash

- The health and nutrition of the caregiver is as important as that of the patient.
- Draw up a list of tasks that facilitates support to the caregiver by different family members, separating caregiving tasks from household chores.
- Allowing the caregiver to take regular breaks, with the help of other family members.
- As a caregiver, in addition to caring for the patient, you should be able to have an occupational activity that distracts you, to avoid stress, but that is compatible with caring for the patient, such as reading, music, that even allows you to get involved.
- The caregiver as well as the patient should exercise, which reduces stress and increases energy.
- Attending support groups for carers
- The caregiver should also seek professional help. Some carers may feel lonely, anxious, guilty, uncomfortable, frightened, overburdened, confused or tired. Their accumulation can lead to a burden of illness.
- The caregiver needs to learn techniques for mobilising the patient and to have a

suitable home environment that facilitates care tasks as safely as possible, to avoid injury.

The aim is to prevent exposure to infections or damage that may affect them.

Promoting family care in home-based care

From the assessment of the family dynamics and with it the reactions and styles of coexistence, external support network, personality, lifestyle, cultural and educational level of the family members; the illness and care of the chronic patient at home can lead to structural alterations of the family evolutionary cycle, alterations to the emotional response, family adaptation with acceptance of the disease process, the patient knows and participates in the prognosis of the disease or the patient and the family do not have a communication process regarding the disease.

C. At the level of patients and caregivers

The caregiver of a patient faces a number of challenges that include not only the knowledge and skill of managing the patient, but also the care of their own health and emotional stability, as the physical and psychological demands of caregiving are often great and have a direct impact on their own quality of life.

Caregivers need to have the knowledge and skills required to provide comprehensive care, not only for the necessary interventions, but for the care to impact on quality of life.

The concept of self-care reinforces the participation of people in their own health care, requires individualisation of care and the involvement of patients and their families in their own care plan.

We can identify four fundamental roles for a home carer (36):

•   Prevention: early detection of situations leading to the biopsychosocial deterioration of the patient.

•   Promotion: identification and optimisation of a patient's existing conditions, as well as the focus on adherence to treatment, generating actions that impact on quality of life.

•   Education: the home caregiver provides information on aspects of care and self-care, teaches demystification of conditions and aspects related to the patients' pathology.

- Assistance: provides support and training to patients for the development of activities of daily living, health care and rehabilitation.

The following are determining factors for a patient with a disability to be supported by a caregiver:

- Age-associated physical factors that occur when the patient is limited in performing simple, everyday activities by natural deterioration of the body due to ageing, degenerative diseases, diminished or total loss of motor, visual or hearing skills.
- Psychological factors generated by: depression, organic mental disorders, memory disturbances.
- Social factors related to: scarce economic resources, inadequate housing for their development, lack of attention from family members.

Once the individual problems have been recognised, it is necessary to associate the care that is required, such as personal care:

- Toilet
- Feeding according to nutritional requirements
- Health monitoring: to provide care necessary for the patient to continue to be active in the social environment.

In the case of an older adult, the most relevant aspects of care are:

- Sleep disorders

- Urinary and Faecal Incontinence

- Immobility

- Balance disorders and dizziness

- Ca^das

- Polypharmacy and self-medication

- General hygiene and care

As aspects to be taken into account in their mental health:

- Isolation

- Mood disorders

- Cognitive disorders

- Dysfunctional grief

The roles of the caregiver include:

- Support and counselling in all activities of daily living.

- Administration of medicines indicated in the medical prescription.
- Assistance during feeding according to the indicated diet.
- General care: general bath in shower or in bed and personal grooming.
- Accident prevention
- Recreational and occupational activities according to the user's possibilities.
- Health promotion and prevention actions
- Administrative procedures related to patient care

Conditions of increased caregiver burden

There are associated factors on the caregiver that create associated risks for the caregiver.

- **Age**: the older you get, the more overburdened you are
- **Gender**: no differentiation, but the focus is on older female caregivers.
- **Number of children**: a greater number of children in the main carer is related to greater overload.
- **Socio-cultural level**: the higher the level of education, the more options for work outside the home and the lower the tendency to burden related to patient care.
- The lower the **economic level**, the higher the overload.
- **Bonding with the sick**: greater burden on spousal caregivers
- **Care time**: the more time available, the less overload caregivers experience.

In conclusion, these bio-psycho-social conditions represent an important risk group on which care and quality of life should be focused, thus making it important to focus on social-health work where it is necessary to develop caregiver support plans, day-care centres, information, communication and psychological support programmes and economic subsidies.

Concerns faced by caregivers

Carers, and in particular if they are the patient's relatives themselves, are confronted with situations such as:

•	Fear of failure as a caregiver: of not being able to do everything the patient requires.

•	Fear of financial problems: because of the expenses related to the care of the family member, especially if the sick person is the main provider in the household.

•	Fear of feeling weak and unable to cope with the additional stress, or of not being able to control the sick person, or of becoming overwhelmed by feelings of pain, anger, resentment or sadness.

•	Fear of their loved one's suffering and feeling limited in what they can do.

•	Fear of performing procedures he/she does not know how to perform or making wrong decisions.

•	Fear of the death of a loved one. When the time of death approaches, sufferers often choose their companion, some prefer to be surrounded, others prefer to be alone.

Based on the development of the spertographic objectives, the following results were obtained:

From the review of documentary evidence related to safe home care practices, in the last five years (2016 to 2020), in national and international databases on the Pubmed, Redalyc and Redcol platforms, using key words:
In English: home care, risks in home care, good safety practices, adverse events.

In English and Portuguese the terms used were: Attention, Environment, Home Care Services, House Calls, Residence Characteristics, Risk Factors, Safety.

By combining the terms: (Home care service) and (Patient safety) and (accident prevention).

A total of 618 articles were obtained, of which 429 were identified prior to 2015 and 189 from the years 2015 to 2020, of which 12 articles refer to adverse events at home and their intervention and 177 to direct topics of care processes. As shown in Figure 2, a total of 12 articles were chosen, six of which correspond to the years

2016 to 2020 and the rest prior to 2015, but were chosen because of their contribution to the research.

In Redalyc, a search was carried out using the keywords Atencion domiciliaria, cuidado domiciliario, home care, home care, patient safety, obtaining 72 articles from the years 2015 to 2020 and 7043 articles from previous years; of the 72 articles identified, we took five that are directly related to adverse events at home, as the remaining 67 refer to other aspects of the care process. See Figure 3.

A search was carried out in Redcol that included 49 repositories of national universities applying the keywords home care, home care, adverse event, finding 246 articles, of which nine were taken related to home care processes, six were discarded as they did not correspond to the defined years and three articles remained which were related to home care processes. See Figure 4.

Figure 2. PUBMED search Figure **3**. REDALYC search

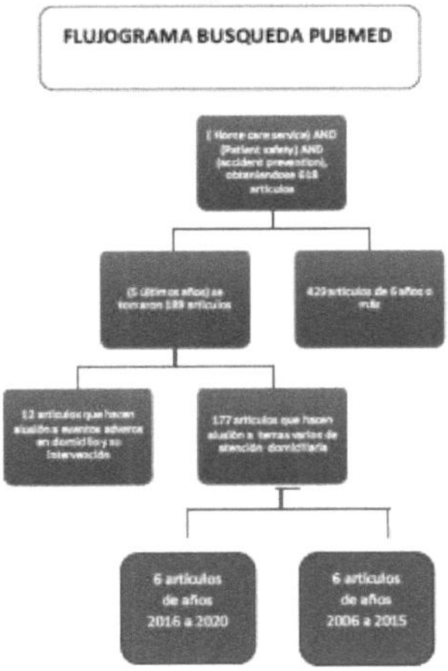

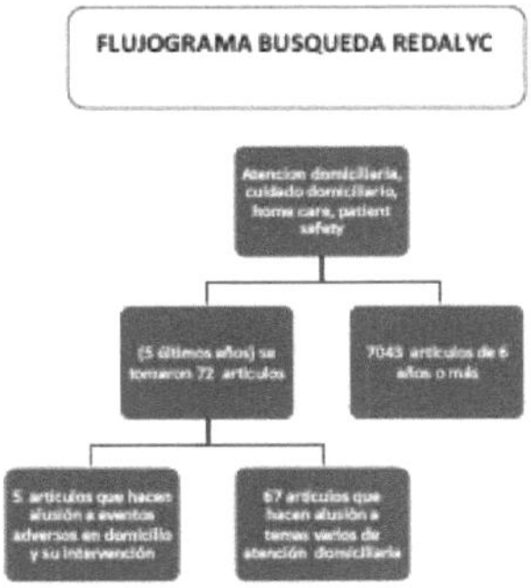

Figure 4. REDCOL search

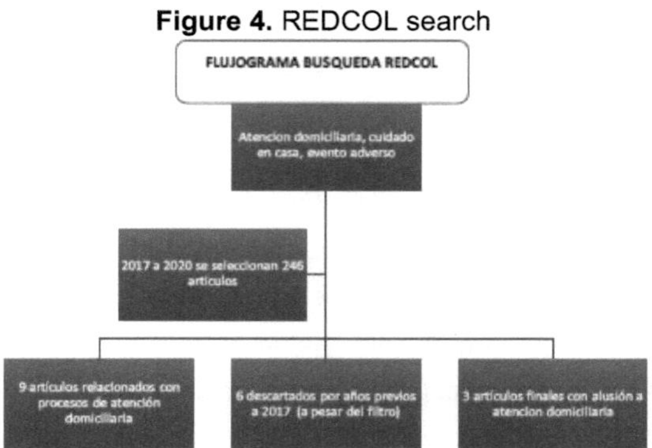

From the Pubmed search we obtained 618 articles; filtering by time period (years 2016 to 2020) we took 189 articles of which we reviewed those that provide recommendations or safe practices to address adverse events in the home, as shown in Figure 2 (and Annex A), we took 12 articles that address risks and events in home care, for the chosen time period and we took specifically the article entitled: "Improving quality and safety in nursing homes and home care: protocol for a mixed-methods research design study to implement a leadership intervention" (19) . This article was selected for the study because its objective, in developing leadership competency and guiding managers in their efforts to advance and improve quality and safety strategies, attitudes and practices vital to their organisations, is close to our objective of identifying risks and events in home care, whose root cause analysis allowed us to propose safe practices to reduce events and intervene in identified risks as a safety strategy in home care.

In terms of the Redalyc search, as shown in Figure 3 (see Annex B), five articles related to critical factors in home care were selected for the study period, such as caregiver, model of care, epidemiological profile, perception of managers, quality of care, mainly.

Of these, the article entitled "Burden of care in caregivers of chronically ill persons in a home hospitalisation programme"(29) was taken as the most important article for the research, taking into account the importance of caregiver burden as a contributory factor in the genesis of adverse events and incidents at home.

From the search carried out on the Redcol platform, as shown in Figure 4 (see Annex C), three articles were prioritised related to quality indicators; review of home care models and relevant aspects for the design of a training programme for caregivers; the article on "knowledge of home care programme models" being of greater relevance for this research as an input element to recognise aspects of the home context and its functioning as important contributing factors in the occurrence of events in the home environment.

2. The following information was obtained from the identification of the adverse events reported in the IPS of low complexity home care during a period of 3 years (2018 to 2020) and their main causes, whose services are provided in three modalities: chronic patient without ventilator, hospitalisation at home and non-oncological palliative care of medium and low complexity, which require management with interdisciplinary support for both the patient and their family, in the process of

disease and outcomes, the following information was obtained.

In the institution a procedure is developed for the identification of adverse events through an application that reaches all staff members, where the report of identified cases is made, then the information is analysed by the patient safety area where the type of event is classified and the head in charge of the programme develops the analysis and defines the respective improvement plan.

Within the identification of adverse events reported by the IPS for the period 2018 to 2020, we obtained the information listed in Table 7.

Table 7. Prioritisation of adverse events in the home-based programme 2018 to 2020

ADVERSE EVENT	Year 2018	Year 2019	Year 2020	Total cases for the 3 years	Percentage of cases
Adverse drug reaction		5			31%
Phlebitis		1	SD	10	18%
Related to surgery or procedures	SD	8	SD	8	15%
Pressure ulcers		SD	SD		13%
Related to Medicines			SD		13%
Events related to non-delivery of Oxygen		SD	SD		5,50%
Inappropriate diagnosis or behaviour					4%
Total events per year					100%

Note. based on the IPS information analysed.

Applying Pareto methodology to prioritise the adverse events reported, as shown in Table 8, we find that the first four adverse events identified correspond to 77% of the cases reported in the period analysed.

Table 8. Prioritisation of adverse events period 2018 to 2020 by Pareto methodology

ADVERSE EVENT	Year 2018	Year 2019	Year 2020	Total cases for the 3 years	Percentage of cases	Cumulative Percentage
Adverse drug reaction		5			31%	31%
Phlebitis		1	SD	10	18%	49%
Related to surgery or procedures	SD	8	SD	8	15%	64%
Pressure ulcers		SD	SD		13%	77%

Note. Based on information from the IPS analysed.

Characterisation of adverse events:

The total population that has received care in the home-based programme of the IPS under study for the years 2018 to 2020, corresponds to 10,822 users, of which 6,508 are women and 4,314 are men.

For the study, we have taken a sample of 40 users who presented any of the four prioritised adverse events, characterised as shown in Table 9 as follows:

Table 9. Characterisation of adverse events

Tipo de evento adverso	Reacción adversa a medicamentos	Flebitis	Postoperatorio o secundario a procedimientos	Úlceras por presión
Género predominante	Femenino	Femenino	Femenino	Femenino
Relación mujer: hombre	12:5	8:2	5:03	1:10
Grupos de edad	4 casos en grupo 21 a 30 años Décadas 30, 50 y 70 años: 3 casos en c/u	3 casos en grupo de 31 a 40 años Décadas 20 y 60 años: 2 casos en c/u	2 casos en menores de 20 años Décadas de 20; 40; 50; 60 y 70 años: 1 caso en c/u	Mayores de 80 años
Diagnósticos de base	Celulitis Infección urinaria Absceso periapical Infección respiratoria	Infección urinaria Celulitis	Parálisis cerebral Esclerosis múltiple Trastorno del desarrollo Infección urinaria Neumonía EPOC	EPOC Demencia Secuelas de evento cerebrovascular Hipertensión

Type of event adverse	Adverse drug reaction	Phlebitis	Postoperative o secondary to procedures	Pressure ulcers
Predominant gender	Female	Female	Female	Female
Relationship woman: man	12:5	8:2	5:03	1:00
Age groups	4 cases in group 21 a 30 years Decades 30s; 50s and 70s years: 3 cases each	3 cases in group of 31 to 40 years Decades 20 y 60 years: 2 cases in each	2 cases in children under 20 years Decades of 20; 40; 50; 60 y 70 years: 1 case each	Over 80 years old
Basic diagnostics	Celu litis Urinary tract infection Periapical abscess Respiratory infection	Urinary tract infection Celu litis	Cerebral palsy Multiple sclerosis Developmental disorder Urinary tract infection Pneumonia COPD	COPD Demen cia Sequelae of cerebrovascular event Hypertension

Note. Based on information from the IPS analysed.

The events related to adverse drug reactions occurred more in the female population (with a female:male ratio of 12:5), mainly in the 21-30 age group with four cases, followed by the 30, 50 and 70 age groups with three cases each. As for the diagnoses related to this event, there were four patients with cellulitis, three with urinary tract infection, one patient with periapical abscess and other cases associated with respiratory infections.

As for phlebitis, there were more cases in females (with a ratio of 8:2), the age group with the highest prevalence was 31-40 years with three cases, and for the 20s and 60s, each with two cases. As for related diagnoses, we found urinary tract infection and cellulitis with four cases each.

For events related to injury to a postoperative patient or secondary to an outpatient procedure (home procedures such as catheter placement), there were more cases in females, with a ratio of 5:3; with a higher prevalence in the under-20 age group (two cases of minors with sequelae of cerebral palsy) and the presence of one case in the 20s, 40s, 50s, 60s and 70s respectively. The most frequent related diagnoses were: cerebral palsy; multiple sclerosis; developmental disorder; urinary tract infection, pneumonia and COPD.

The event of pressure ulcers is mainly recorded in women over 80 years of age, with diagnoses of COPD, dementia, hypertension and sequelae of cardiovascular events.

2.1 Identifying and managing risks in the IPS

Within the identification of risks within the IPS, there is a global procedure that includes: risk identification, analysis, risk assessment, with which the inherent risks are established and subsequently the identification and definition of causes and controls with which the residual risks are defined. The controls defined are preventive (they prevent the occurrence of an event) and corrective (they do not prevent the event, but allow the situation to be dealt with once it occurs).

The IPS has a process for prioritising adverse events in the home care programme, which for the years 2018, 2019 and 2020 are described as a prioritisation matrix for inherent and residual risks.

In relation to the inherent risks, as shown in Table 10, the following were prioritised as high: non-adherence to guidelines with 67% compliance for an established target of 75%; patient satisfaction with 88% compliance and a target of 95%; and re-admission of patients to hospital with a deviation of more than 2.5% for the year 2019. Moderate risks were found to be: the presence of new pressure ulcers during the stay in the home programme, non-control of diabetic patients, non-control of hypertensive patients, infection of patients treated at home and poorly completed medical records.

Table 10. Matrix of inherent risks and their controls, years 2018 to 2020

BEHAVIOUR OF THE MAIN INCIDENTS IN HOME-BASED CARE 2018 TO 2020 INHERENT RISK MATRIX						
RISK	GOAL OF THE INDICA DOR	2018	2019	2020	RISK CLASSIFICATION	CONTROLS
No giia adberecia eв BteacioB domiciliary	75*	63,30*	68,50*	67,70*	ALTO	Training on clinical practice guidelines and access to them Annual review of the morbidity of processes Feedback to doctors on deviations detected during the audit.
Satisfaction of the	941	315;	73*	88,50*	ALTO	Shift configuration of 6 to 8 hours max. Humanisation Programme Training Registration of complaints, claims and suggestions Delivery of the process folder (3 leaflets education, general recommendations, etc.) acute patient y chronic patient)
paciettes a bospitalizaBility	2.50*	1.16%	2,50*	0,30*	ALTO	External o internal trainings Periodic medical check-ups according to pathologies Patient identification protocol Adverse event or incident report Registration of complaints, claims and suggestions
Pressure ulcers - "you were during the	2/1000 attention	0.86	0,1	0	MODERATE	Educating the caregiver workshop Adverse event or incident report

stat es the process of aBtiBcation	is					Follow-up of hospital readmissions
No control of diabetic patients?	60*	67,30*	78,30*	75,30*	MODERATE	Training on the management of chronic diabetic patients Training on the management of chronic diabetic patients Review report on avoidable causes of hospitalisation Training on clinical management protocol
patients seen	3/ 1.000 is	0	0.2	0,2	MODERATE	Educating the caregiver workshop
Non-control of biperteaceous patients	80*	86,305;	82,30*	30,30*	MODERATE	Adverse event reporting o Incident Chronic patient management training Chronic patient management training Review preventable causes of hospitalisation report
Mai diligence of the Clinical History	85*	82,70*	32,70*	88,50*	MODERATE	Training in the use of the HC application (induction). Internal trainings Feedback to the doctors on the deviations detected in the audit.

Note: Based on IPS risk management information.

Once the causes and controls for the inherent risks had been analysed, we checked the residual risk matrix, see Table 11, where no high risks were identified and moderate risks were identified as delays in patient care at home, cancellation of visits due to institutional causes, patient dissatisfaction, and low risks were classified as follows, The following are classified as low risks: no control of diabetic patients, no control of hypertensive patients, re-admission of patients to hospitalisation, new pressure ulcers during the stay, in the process of home care, poor completion of the medical history, infection of patients attended and delay in the administration of medicines during the service, to which control plans should be applied.

Table 11. Matrix of residual risks and their controls for years 2018 to 2020

RISK	INDICATOR TARGET	BEHAVIOUR OF THE MAIN INCIDENTS HOME CARE 2018 TO 2020 RESIDUAL RISK MATRIX				CAUSES	CONTROLS
		2018	2019	2020	- The tIESCO		
Patient satisfaction; attended;	34%	31%	73%	88,50%	MODERATE	Fatigue, work overload, staff turnover, non-adherence to the humanisation programme, ineffective humanisation programme.	Humanisation Programme Training Strengthen the humane treatment of health professionals Registration of complaints, claims and suggestions;
No patient control; diabetic;	60%	67,30%	78.30%	75,30%	UNDER	Lack of adherence in the management of clinical practice guidelines Lack of patient adherence to medical therapy Insufficient installed capacity/ demand	Training; on patient management; chronic diabetic Training; on patient management; chronic diabetic Review cause report; of avoidable hospitalisation;
No control of patient; hypertensive;		86.30%	82.30%	30.30%	UNDER	Lack of adherence in the management of clinical practice guidelines Lack of patient adherence to medical therapy Insufficient installed capacity/ demand	Training; on patient management; chronic Training; on patient management; chronic Review cause report; of avoidable hospitalisation;
Re-admission of patient; to hospitalisation	2.50%	1,16%	2,50%	0,30%	UNDER	Patient's decision/miscommunication failure (non-adherence to guidelines) Decompensation of the underlying pathology Failure to schedule the professional within the timeframe established by the process Error in patient identification	Delivery of the process folder (3 leaflets; education, general recommendations; acute patient and chronic patient) Training; external; or internal; Medical check-ups; periodically according to pathology; Patient identification protocol Report of the adverse event or incident Register of complaints, claims and suggestions;
Ulcer; new pressure ulcer; during stay in the home care process	2/1000 attention;	0,86	0.1	0	UNDER	Decompensation of the underlying pathology	Workshop educating the caregiver Reporting the adverse event o incident Follow-up re-admission; hospital;
Mai medical record filling	85%	82.70%	32.70%	88,50%	UNDER	Non-professional scheduling in the; time; established; by the process	Training in the use of the HC application (induction) Internal training; Feedback to the; physician; of the; deviation; detected; in audit
Patient infection; attended;	3/1.000 attentions;	0	0.2	0.2	UNDER	Lack of education of primary caregiver since active search Unsuitable caregiver	Training on clinical management protocol Caregiver education workshop Adverse event or incident report
Delay in the administration of medication; during the home care service - Proportion of adverse events related to the administration of medication;		0,08%	0.03%	0.02%	UNDER	Lack of training in the use of the medical history application. Lack of training in the; criteria; of measurement in the compilation of the dynamic history. Lack of commitment	Medication Reconciliation Protocol - Medication Management Guide. Registration in dynamic history of novelty Audit to note; of nursing Adverse event or incident report

Note: Based on IPS risk management information.

Improvement actions identified in the programme of the institution analysed:

- Strengthening the reporting culture

- Training for programme staff.

- Identification of the causes that generate adverse events, as well as risk characterisation.

- Cohort follow-up to assess non-adherence to medical treatment, which leads to complications and user dissatisfaction.

- Adjustment to administrative procedures that impact on patient care.

2.2 Risk analysis of the home-based care process provided by the IPS in study (October 2021)

Through the implementation of the FMEA model methodology, three professionals from the IPS were convened: the head doctor of the programme, the medical assistant and the physical therapist, with whom we proceeded to:

- Verify the steps or phases that make up this care process.

- The main **failure modes** occurring at each stage of the process were identified with the help of programme professionals.
- Possible causes were identified for each phase
- The possible effects caused by the identified failures were obtained by consensus of the group of professionals.
- With the help of pre-established matrices previously verified by the participants, we proceeded to rate: probability, severity and ability to detect failures.
- The risk probability index is calculated for each phase and for the entire home care process.

Scope of the process analysed:

It starts with the so-called nurse screening phase in the active search for patients, and ends with the procedure or discharge phase of the programme, in total 15 phases.

Results

The risks affecting the 15 phases identified in the home care process, which the IPS offers today, were analysed.

Of the home care process analysed, the following were prioritised as phases or procedures **with the highest probability** of risk:

Rated as "Very High Probability" with a score of 9- 10/10

1- Continuity of treatment with a probability of 10/10
2- Chronic patient care with a 10/10 chance of success.
3- Delivery of patient report with a probability of 10/10
4- Exit with a probability of 10/10

5- Referral to rehabilitation group with a probability of 9/10

6- Interdisciplinary assessment with a probability of 9/10

In terms of the phases or procedures defined **with the greatest severity**, the following were identified as "Catastrophic risks" with a rating of 9-10/10:

1- Referral by out-patient or emergency physician to home care with severity of 10/10

2- Care in palliative programme with a severity rating of 9/10

The following procedures or phases of the process were rated as **major severity** risk with a rating of 6 to 8/10, ask

1- Doctor's rating of the programme with a value of 8/10

2- Home hospitalisation with a value of 8/10

3- Chronic patient care with 8/10

4- Interdisciplinary assessment with a value of 8/10

5- Treatment plan with a value of 8/10

6- Referral to rehabilitation group with a rating of 7/10

7- Home care planning with a value of 6/10

8- Home care by the appropriate professional with a value of 6/10

9- Continuity of treatment with a value of 6/10

In terms of the **probability of detecting risks**, it was possible to prioritise:

With a risk detection probability rating of "Moderate" and a score of 7 to 8/10 the following process steps/procedures ask

1- Rating by nurse in active search with a rating of 8/10

2- Referral by emergency physician or outpatient physician to the home programme at a value of 8/10

3- Palliative programme with a value of 8/10

4- Home care planning with a value of 7/10

5- Attention by the professional concerned with a value of 7/10

According to the global calculation **of the risk probability index**, it was possible to prioritise the procedures or phases of this process from the highest to the lowest risk, ask

1- Referral by emergency physician and outpatient physician to the home programme with 640/1000

2- Palliative care programme at a value of 360/1000

3- Rating per nurse in active search with 256/1000

4- Referral to rehabilitation group with 252/1000

5- Home-based care planning with 252/1000

6- Home care by appropriate professional with 252/1000

With the information obtained from applying the FMEA model, it was suggested that a "control plan" be drawn up, giving priority to procedures that were identified as being of greater severity or probability, strengthening the control barriers in the procedures prioritised by detection capacity.

3. With regard to the characterisation of the home care experience and its main risks from the point of view of patients, carers and treating professionals, guided interviews were conducted and the following findings were obtained:

3.1. Have the professionals providing your home care explained anything to you about safe care practices?

83% of the respondents were explained how to prevent risks, but in addition 50% of the respondents expressed that they have been explained what are safe practices and what are risks.

3.2. Do you remember if at any time during your home care, any of the professionals who cared for you explained to you how to prevent risks that may occur during home care?

66% of respondents said they have been told about the risk of damage from medication and for 33% of respondents they have been told about other risks, such as the risk of bedsores and the risk of "desaturation".

3.3. What risks do you identify that you may face during home care by any of the home care team?

66% indicated the risk of falls; 33% expressed the risk of infections, but in addition 66% added risk related to medication use.

3.4. Do you consider that the recommendations given to you by the home care professionals need to be improved?

50% of the respondents considered that something written, such as a user manual, should be annexed, and 16% expressed that a query should be added as a control.

3.5. Do you believe that the risks of injury or damage that occur to patients during home care are the responsibility of?

50% of respondents considered it to be a shared responsibility between patient, caregiver, health care team and HPS; 33% felt it was the responsibility of the patient and caregiver; 16% of respondents argued that it was the responsibility of the health care team.

3.6. How do you or your caregiver experience these good practices during home care, how have they helped you?

All respondents reported that they listen to them, learn from them and put them into practice, but 83% felt that it has also helped them to avoid further consequences.

3.7. For the risks you have experienced during home care, what good practices do you consider to take into account?

For 100% the main risk identified is the care with the handling of medicines, but also for 50% the care related to diet, cures and falls is important; 16% also expressed the importance of care related to the skin.

3.8. How does the health care team, as a patient or caregiver, teach you about good safety practices in home care?

66% reported that they are only explained verbally; 33% that they are taught with a primer or video or explained through examples.

3.9. What do you propose to improve the home care programme, to be taken into account as good care practices?

50% of respondents thought that they would like to have fewer administrative procedures, especially for medicines and more services at home (vaccinations and specialised consultations in some cases of bedridden patients); 33% thought that they would like to have more staff available for home care and 17% thought that they would like to be given more explanations in this respect.

3.10. In your experience, who do you consider to be most at risk during your home care, rate the highest risk with 5, the lowest risk with 4, 3 or 2 and the lowest risk with 1, in the items below:

For 66%, the priority is given to risks due to medicines, then to the availability of professionals, followed by administrative procedures, with equipment and the risks inherent in the home facilities being considered the least risky, with the latter insisting that the risks are already identified and protected against.

Figura 5.   Summary of user and carer surveys

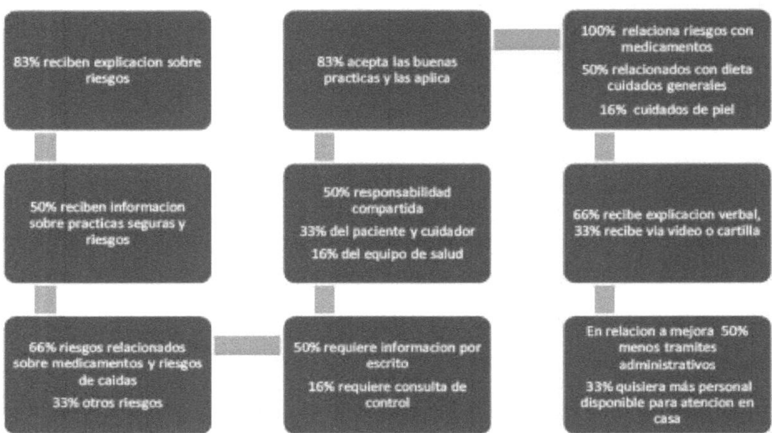

5.2. With regard to the results of the survey of professionals in the home care programme:

3.2.1 Knowledge of "Good patient safety practices in home care" guidelines

29% of the respondents represented by one general practitioner and one nursing assistant reported not knowing guidelines on good patient safety practices in home care, all other professionals said they did.

3.2.2. As to the source of information on safety in home care with which you are familiar:

In response to this positive response, 57% (a doctor, a social worker, a nurse and a nurse's aide) said they knew them from the IPS where they currently work and 43% (a doctor, a nurse and a nurse's aide) said they knew them from another institution where they worked.

3.2.3. To the question: Have you received extra-institutional guidelines on security in home care and from which source?

71% reported not having received any guidelines, while 14% (one doctor) of respondents said they were aware of international guidelines and 14% (one doctor)

were aware of national guidelines.

3.2.4. The organisation where you work promotes training in good safe practices in home-based care.
100% responded in the affirmative.

3.2.5. ^ Considering that if training is promoted in your institution, you wonder how it is promoted?

85% indicated that they are trained by the same institution, only the social worker stated that she did not receive the training from the same institution where she works.

3.2.6. Regarding the training you receive from the institution where you work, you consider that this training was:

56% of the training was specific to good practice in home care safety, corresponding to a doctor, therapist and nursing assistants; 14% reported that the training had not been specific to safe practice in home care and 30% (social worker and nurse) indicated that they had only been trained in event and incident reporting.

3.2.7 When asked how do you inform patients and carers about safe home care practices?

57% (nurse, therapist and assistants) responded that they demonstrate with examples or are given lectures and for 14% (nurse practitioner) they indicated that tasks were left to patients and carers.

3.2.8 When asked what are the main risks identified in home-based care, the respondents identified several risks, ask

71% (doctor, nurse, therapist and auxiliary) indicated that the main risks are related to medication; 43% (doctor, therapist and auxiliary) expressed that they are infections and 57% (social worker, doctors and nurse practitioner) stated that the main risks are related to skin care.

3.2.9 ^How do you evaluate the impact of good security practices?

The two doctors (28%) responded that it is done through home care safety indicators; one assistant (14%) said it is evaluated by rating what patients and carers have learned and the social worker responded that it is done through the evaluation of events and incidents; 57% (doctor, nurse, therapist and one assistant) responded that it is done through the evaluation of the knowledge of health professionals.

3.2.10 ^In the implementation of good safety practices in home care and your suggestion to make them more effective?

The social worker, doctors, nurse and therapist (71%) responded that safe practices should be made exclusively for home care; while one auxiliary (14%) considered that they should be included in the training plan and another auxiliary that they should be evaluated frequently.

3.2.11 ^What do you consider to be the main impact of implementing good home care safety practices in your institution?

The social worker, doctors, therapist and assistants (85%) felt that there are fewer injuries to patients, and the nurse and therapist (15%) felt that this is reflected in the rating of health professionals.

3.2.12 ^Is it prioritised which adverse events have been improved through the application of good safety practices?

One physician and nursing assistants (42%) indicated that infection-related adverse events have been improved; for nursing assistants (28%) risks related to falls were impacted and 100% of respondents agree that skin care-related events can be improved.

3.2.13 Do you know of any manual or instructions on home care safety in the institution where you work?

The social worker, the doctors and the nurse (42%) considered that, yes, it exists, but it is not specific for home-based care.

3.2.14 ^If the training plan could include good safety practices in home care, prioritise some of the proposed topics?

The nurse, the therapist and the assistant (45%) prioritised what good home care safety practices are and how they are implemented, while for the therapist and the assistant (28%) they considered that evaluation of the correct implementation of good home care safety practices should be prioritised and for the doctor and the nurse (28%), the next priority is related to information to patients and caregivers, while for a doctor (14%) how to evaluate the correct implementation of good home care practices was a priority.

3.2.15 How do you consider from your professional experience that the implementation of good safety practices in home care could contribute to:

The social worker, the two doctors, the therapist and the two assistants (85%) considered that it would help to avoid harm to patients; the social worker and the nurse (28%) considered that it would help to maintain the confidence of the patient and his family and the social worker considered that it would also help to avoid legal risks.

Figura 6.   Summary of interviews with professionals

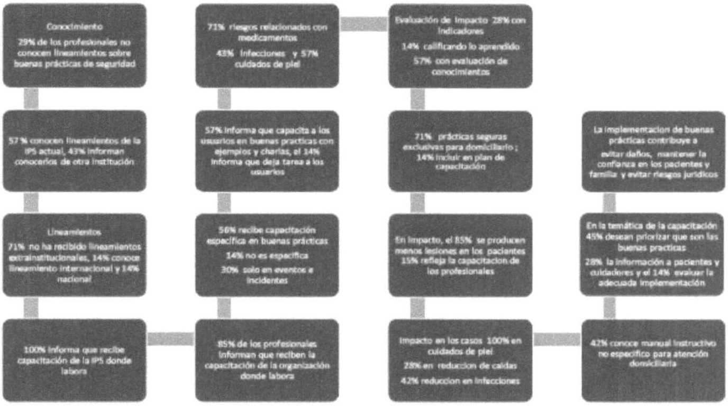

Analysing the results of this survey of professionals in the home care programme as a whole, some perceived risks were identified as shown in Table 12.

Table 12. Percentage of prioritisation of risks in home care by surveyed professionals

	Identified Risks	Percentage of respondents' opinion
1	There are no safe practices specific for home care	71%
	Risks related to the use of medicines	71%
	Risks related to care of the skin	5//o

Note: Information from the survey of professionals.

4. With respect to the evaluation of the applicability, scope and results of the implementation of the existing guidelines for the prevention of adverse events and unsafe care in a low complexity home care service, the following results were obtained from the surveys applied:

6.1 What guidelines on good safety practice in home care are you aware of?

The Ministry Kderes, IPS manager, Hder of home-based programme and Hder of patient safety (80%) responded that they are aware of the instructional packages published by the Ministry of Health, which are not expected for home-based care.

6.2 Safe practice guidelines available to the organisation you represent?

The IPS manager and the Hder of the safety programme (40%) responded that they adapt the good practices presented by the Ministry of Health that apply at the household level; while 60% do not know, do not answer.

6.3 How do these guidelines in practice contribute to improving safety in care?

For the IPS manager and for the head of home care (40%) events and incidents are reduced or mitigated; for the head of patient safety (20%) the aim is to minimise risks; for the Secretary's Hder (20%) they improve safety for patients and professionals and for the Ministry's Hder (20%) the remaining practices are not exclusive to home care, processes are promoted to ensure good practice in different areas.

6.4 What adjustments do you suggest to improve good practice in home care?

The Ministry of Health Hder and the IPS manager (40%) reported the need for ongoing training of health personnel; the Ministry of Health Hder and the head of the home-based programme (40%) considered that evidence-based medicine guidelines should be taken into account; the head of patient safety (20%) indicated that the particularities of the context should be taken into account; the IPS manager and the quality manager of the ministry (40%) considered that the caregiver should be taken into account; the IPS manager (20%) considered that the patient and family should be integrated, as well as investment in technology to improve the implementation of safe practices.

6.5 What risks justify good practice in home care?

The IPS manager and the head of patient safety (40%) indicated that care-associated infections and drug-related events are evident; the Hder of the Ministry of Health (20%) explained that risks are not having expected guidelines and lack of control by the EPS; the Hder of the Ministry was of the opinion that all events, risks and failure modes warrant analysis and intervention.

6.6 Evidence in the organisation you represent of measuring safe practices?

The IPS manager explained that they carry out internal audits to assess compliance with home safety guidelines in patients and relatives; for the Hder of the Ministry of Health there is monitoring of priority processes but nothing specific for home care;

the head of patient safety said that the risks are known and only their materialisation is monitored; the Hder of the Ministry explained that there are safe practices in hospitals and not at home and the head of home services omitted information.

6.7 How to involve patients and families in the development of these good practices?

For the IPS manager and the patient safety Hder, the participation of the patient and his/her family is fundamental; for the Hder of the Secretary of Health and for the patient safety Hder, sensitisation, training and training of caregivers is required; for the head of the home care service, active participation in decision-making in treatment is important.

6.8 How does the institution where you work assess the degree of understanding of safe practices in patients and caregivers?

In 40% of the institutions surveyed (territorial entities), they reported that there is no evaluation; for the 40% corresponding to EPS and IPS representatives the evaluation of these practices is very low and only for the head of patient safety the evaluation is done with workshops for caregivers and evaluation of process effectiveness indicators.

6.9 Difficulties identified for the implementation of safe home care practices?

For the representative of the Secretary of Health, neither the caregiver nor the family are well prepared for the provision of care at home; for the national entity this scope is not evaluated; for the manager of the IPS the high turnover of health personnel does not facilitate it; for the Hder of the home programme the difficulty of access to some sites and for the Hder of patient safety the lack of adherence of personnel to institutional guidelines are the main difficulties for the application of safe practices in home care.

6.10   How are the guidelines for good practice in home care applied?

The Ministry's Hder, the IPS manager and the patient safety Hder were of the opinion that the good practice guidelines are the official document, which has been adopted by the institutions and is applied to the care model; the Hder of the Health Secretariat indicated that there are no expected guidelines for home care and 20% do not know, no answer.

6.11   For the respondents, are these safe practices specially adapted for home-based care or not and why?

Neither for the Ministry, nor for the representative of the Territorial Secretariat, are these practices expected for home-based care; the manager of the IPS reported that they are adapted to the home environment, while neither for the Kderes of the home-based programme, nor for the security Hder, are these guidelines expected for home-based care.

6.12   Positive indicators of safe practice in home care?

For the Ministry and for the Territorial Secretariat they are not contemplated or are not expected for the home environment; for the management of the IPS this measurement of indicators is starting this year; while for Hder of the home programme and for Hder of safety the most important positive indicator is that of adverse drug reactions.

6.13   Has there been any learning in the institutions you represent about the implementation or evaluation of safe practices in home-based care?

For the local authorities, there is nothing expected for home-based care; for the IPS, only 20% of the respondents felt that guidelines and guidelines have been identified that are not very expected for home-based care.

6.14   Has your organisation considered the inclusion of safe home care practices in its training plan?

For local and regional authorities, this is not expected, while for IPS representatives, it is expected.

6.15   How has this training been reflected in good home care practices?

In territorial entities it was found that there is no measurement, while for the IPS, 20% is reflected by the increase in adverse event reports; for 20% by the decrease in clinical outcome indicators and for 20% it impacts the knowledge of collaborators in basic principles such as safety goals.

6.16   When implementing safety practices in home-based care, what results do you find most relevant, please rate?

The participants prioritised with 100% the prevention of injuries to the patient; for the referent of the Ministry, the referent of the Departmental Health Secretariat, for the Hder of the domiciliary programme and for the Hder of patient safety, the prevention of consequences for the family; for the referent of the Secretariat, for the manager and for the Hder of the domiciliary service, the avoidance of cost overruns and for the referent of the Ministry and the Hder of safety, it is about preserving the patient's trust in the institution and with 80% the least relevant result is the avoidance of health risks.

6.17   How to identify the experience of patients and their families in implementing safe home care practices?

100% reported that they have not identified this experience in patients and their relatives and only in the IPS they are in this process and expect to identify it from this year onwards.

In relation to the questions asked in the surveys of the system's Kderes, we found the following aspects in summary:

Figura 7.   Summary of surveys carried out on System Kderes

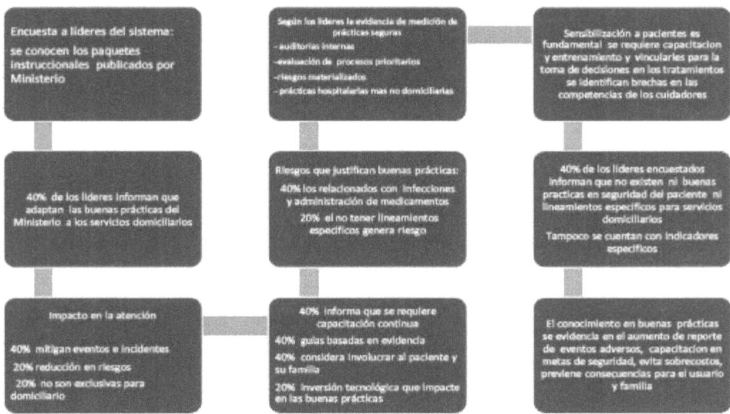

Based on the results of the survey of health system referents, it was possible to prioritise the most evident risks as shown in Table 13.

Table 13. Percentage of prioritisation of home care risks in health system referents surveyed.

	Identified risks	Percentage of respondents' opinions
1	Risk of care-associated infections Risks related to lack of more active patient and family involvement	
	Risks of applying non-specific home care practices	20%
	Risks related to lack of communication and training of caregivers and patients	20%

Note. Based on Hderes survey.

49

Chapter 5

Discussion

Work in Spain (ENEAS; APEAS) and in Latin America (IBEAS; AMBEAS) has focused on the investigation of events and incidents at the inpatient and outpatient levels, but very little work has concentrated on the risks of home care.

From the international and national bibliographic search, it was possible to identify that events are mainly analysed and, to a lesser extent, incidents at home, all of which are adjusted to a model of care and environmental conditions of developed countries, with resources and greater opportunities than our Latin American countries.

For this reason, this research has focused on identifying the most relevant risk factors in home care, under a "sui generis" Colombian health system, in the patient's living environment, in developing countries, with special emphasis on the analysis of the causes that favour the occurrence of the main events and incidents in home care.

From the review of the database of a low complexity home care IPS, it was identified that the emphasis of the report and its analysis is focused on adverse events but not on incidents. This has led to some irregularity in reporting and poor performance in the analysis of the causes, which has become a limiting factor in the establishment of more effective improvement actions.

Therefore, it is necessary to strengthen the culture of incident identification and reporting, as well as the analysis of the causes, in order to propose interventions adjusted to the reality of home-based care, so as to have specific safe practices and procedures for this type of care.

With regard to the experiences of patients, carers and professionals attending the home care service, very relevant aspects were identified related to the lack of specific training for carers, the lack of effectiveness of the education received by patients, as well as the great importance of administrative risks related to the delivery of medicines and authorisations, which become relevant contributing factors in the occurrence of events and incidents in home care.

It should be noted that most of the patients surveyed had a caregiver, but there are some who, according to their family conditions, may not have one; therefore, the proposal suggests that the basic criterion for this type of care should be the existence of a caregiver, whether technical or non-technical, who is responsible for the care of the patient, guaranteeing adherence to the treatment.

The Ministry of Social Protection and the Ministry of Health's guidelines emphasise the lack of expected guidelines that guarantee patient safety in home care; although it is true that the mandatory standards, such as the habilitation, mention the extramural care provided at home and some basic criteria for this service, it is very limited in terms of safe practices and procedures; This proposal aims to strengthen safe practices in low complexity home care, proposing some tools to providers, patients and caregivers to identify and manage the main risks of this type of care.

It is also proposed that the Ministry of Social Protection and the local authorities should take into account, as their own functions of direction, surveillance and control of the system, that home care should be conceived as a very significant part of the comprehensive care that the system should offer to users.

For administrators to include risk management within the benefit plan that is specific to home care and not as a part of outpatient care or as an extension of inpatient care.

Finally, as an integrating proposal we want to present safe practices and procedures, where home care is taken into account as part of the integral care of the benefit plan, with minimum criteria to guarantee safe care for the patient at home; with a care model focused on patient safety; emphasising at the provider level where safe practices are proposed for the first causes of adverse events that most affect care in this service.

Finally, a contribution for patients and caregivers to empower them and reduce the risks of events and incidents, based on minimum practices to be considered when receiving a home care service.

Conclusions

From this research, and once the objectives have been met, we can conclude the following aspects:

There is very little literature found at international and national level related to safety in home care and few specific proposals for safe home care practices and procedures.

Given that most of the lessons learned in patient safety come from inpatient care and moderately from outpatient care, further study of risks in home care is needed to document safe practices in the home such as those proposed as a result of this research.

Recognising the lack of expected normative guidelines for home-based care, it is necessary to work on the development of expected public policy for home-based care and for the safety of home-based care, to be adopted in a compulsory manner by each and every one of the actors of the General Health Security System.

With this proposal for safe practices in home care we want to open the door to research and development of safe practices and procedures, their implementation and improvement for Colombia and for any country working for the quality of home care.

As a product of the development of this proposal for safe practices in low complexity home care, we can recommend:

1- Promote further research into the prevention of adverse events and incidents in different settings, mainly in outpatient and home settings, given the particular conditions of our health system as opposed to other health systems in other countries.

2- It is of great importance to study adverse events and incidents in the patient care environment before proposing adaptations of work, based on specific risk environments and conditions specific to each care process.

3- To take into account the experience of users and their families when analysing the quality of care and in particular home care, where the patient and his or her carer are the main axis of the care process.

4- It is suggested that in the Colombian health care model, special importance should be given to home-based care, given the trend towards outsourcing that exists today in health care worldwide.

5- It is suggested that the minimum conditions that must be met in a home-based care process be incorporated into the national security policy and in the qualification criteria, in order to work towards their fulfilment.

6- We hope that this proposal will motivate research into safe practices and procedures in different care settings, in order to work towards continuous quality improvement in health care.

Bibliography

1. Ministerio de Salud y Proteccion Social- Calidad de atencion en salud- Seguridad del paciente- 2010

2. Ministry of Health and Social Protection - Guidelines for the implementation of the patient safety policy. 2008

3. Sanchez D- Camelo - Giraldo Clara Prevalence of adverse events in the home care programme. University Foundation of the Andean Area. Bogota 2014-2015

4. Sanchez M, Fuentes G. Technical management of home care programmes. Rev CES Salud Publica. 2016

5. Law 100 of 1993. Official Journal 41.148 of 23 December 1993.

6. Ministry of Health. Resolution 3100 of 2019

7. Ministry of Health. Resolution 2626 of 2019. MAITE territorial integrated care model.

8. National Health System Quality Agency (2008). Estudio APEAS: Estudio sobre la seguridad de los pacientes en atencion primaria de salud. Ministry of Health and Consumer Affairs Publications Centre.

9. Pan American Health Organization. Results of the PAHO/WHO AMBEAS study: Protocol to determine the frequency, characteristics and avoidability of Adverse Events (AE) in patients in outpatient care in Latin America and the Caribbean.

10. Ministry of Health. Lineamientos implementacion poHtica nacional de seguridad del paciente. Bogota November 2008

11. Ministry of Health. Good practice guide for patient safety in health care. 2010

12. Buedo P- Salas M. Atencion de la salud en domicilio, aportes desde la bioetica. Revista latinoamericana de Bioetica, vol 19, num 2. 2019. Universidad militar nueva granada

13. Baquero-Molina, N. Lineamientos para el Programa de Atencion Domiciliaria. Subsecretana de Servicios de Salud y Aseguramiento; 2017.

14. Ministry of Social Protection. Resolution No. 1446 of 2006. Technical annex to the quality information system, quality monitoring indicators.

15. Nathalie Mockli , Michael Simon , Carla Meyer-Massetti , Sandrine Pihet , Roland Fischer , Matthias Wachter , Christine Serdaly , and Franziska Zuniga Factors associated with home care coordination and quality of care: a research protocol for a national multicentre cross-sectional study. 2021

16. Johannessen T, Ree E, Str0mme T, Aase I, Bal R, Wiig S. Design and pilot testing of a leadership intervention to improve quality and safety in nursing homes

and home care (the SAFE-LEAD intervention) 2019.

17. Maria nelcy munoz astudillo, Liliana Torres Bedoya, Luz Yaneth Lenis, Jonathan Morales Giraldo, Yeferson Cano Diaz, Daniela Londono Arcila Percepcion de trabajadores sobre la cultura de seguridad del paciente en una empresa de salud. 2019

18. Siri Wiig , Eline Ree , Terese Johannessen , Torunn Str0mme , Marianne Storm , Ingunn Aase , Berit Ullebust , Elisabeth Holen-Rabbersvik , Line Hurup Thomsen , Anne Torhild Sandvik Pedersen , Hester van de Bovenkamp , Roland Bal , and Karina Aase Improving quality and safety in nursing homes and home care: the study protocol of a mixed-methods research design to implement a leadership intervention. 2018

19. Catherine E. Tong, Joanie Sims-Gould, and Anne Martin-Matthews
Types and patterns of safety concerns in home care: client and family caregiver perspectives. 2016

20. Sarah Bamgbaden, Valorie Dearmon Fall prevention for older adults receiving home health care. 2016

21. Margherita C. Labson Adapting the Joint Commission's Seven Fundamentals for a Safe and Effective Transition from Care to Home. 2015

22. Lena Swedberg , Eva Hammar Chiriac, Lena Tornkvist and Ingrid Hylander From risky home care to safer home care: health care assistants striving to overcome lack of training, supervision and support. 2013

23. Marilyn T Macdonald, Ariella Lang, Janet Storch, Lynn Stevenson,Tanya Barber, Kristine Iaboni, and Susan Donaldson Examining markers of safety in home care using the international classification for patient safety. 2013

24. Paul Massotti; Mary Ann Mc Coll; Michael Green Adverse events experienced by home care patients: a scoping review of the literature. 2010

25. Ariella Lang, Marilyn Macdonald, Jan Storch, Kari Elliott, Lynn Stevenson, Helene Lacroix, Susan Donaldson, Serena Corsini-Munt, Farraminah Francis and Cherie Geering Curry Safety perspectives on home-based care for clients, family members, caregivers and paid providers. 2009

26. Keir G. Johnson Adverse events among Winnipeg home care clients. 2006

27. Pinzon-Rocha, Mana L.; Galvis-Lopez, Clara R.; Vacca-Casanova, Ana B. Perception of managers of home-based care programmes in the department of Meta. 2019

28. Gonzalez Rodriguez, Raidel Calidad de la atención medica dirigida a adultos

mayores fragiles. 2018

29. Rodriguez Marin, Jorge Eliecer; Valencia Rico, Claudia Liliana; Gonzalez Franco, Stefania; de la Pava Munoz, Karen Carga de cuidado en cuidadores de personas con enfermedad cronica pertenecientes a un programa de hospitalizacion en casa (Manizales, Colombia). 2018

30. Pavlovic, Andres; Calderon, Oscar; Munoz, Eduardo; Carcamo, Marcela; Triana, Jenny; Morales, Karen Descripcion de los pacientes mayores de 60 anos ingresados al programa de hospitalizacion domiciliaria del complejo asistencial. 2016

31. Jaen-Posada, Juan Sebastian; Gutierrez-Gutierrez, Elena Valentina; Cortes-Zapata, Sebastian Epidemiological profile of patients in the home hospitalisation service of a level three institution in the Aburra Valley, 2015.

32. Castilla Amaya, L. V. Review of home care models for older adult patients with chronic and terminal illnesses from the point of view of adherence to treatment and quality of life. 2020

33. Lozano Zamora, A. M., & Beltran Medina, A. M. Relevant aspects for the design of a training programme aimed at the primary caregiver of chronic patients. 2019

34. Puchi, C., Paravic Klijn, T., & Salazar, A. Indicadores de calidad de la atención en salud en hospitalizacion domiciliaria: revisión integradora. 2018

35. Franco Corso, J. Diseno de PoKticas Publicas 3 A Edicion, accessed 9 November 2021. Available at https://www.casadellibro.com/ebook-diseno-de-politicas-publicas-3a-edicion-ebook/9786079722975/11614271

36. Role, functions and profile of the home caregiver. National University of La Plata. https://unlp.edu.ar/frontend/media/12/27612/1b0316aa34127fc82a3fd1f85fec00a1.pdf

Annex A. Safe practice chart for low complexity home care.

Safe practices are proposed for the four prioritised adverse events in home care:

1. Adverse drug reactions

Identifying adverse drug reaction as the first cause of adverse events, which corresponds to one of the problems related to the use of medicines (PRUM).

General objective

To minimise risks and possible adverse drug reactions that may occur during the administration of medicines to home care patients by generating strategies that ensure the correct use of medicines with the least risk and the best results.

Specific objectives

• To identify the active failures that exist during the process of administering medicines in home care.
• Identify contributory factors inherent to the patient, the task and technology, the health care team and the patient's care environment.
• Define the main latent failures that occur during the administration of medicines that may lead to the occurrence of adverse drug reactions.
• Establish safety barriers to prevent active failures, contributory factors or possible latent failures that may favour the occurrence of adverse drug reactions in home care.

Outreach

This package applies to the care of patients at home, under the care of a health institution, through a home care team.

Applying the problem-based approach methodology, we will have:

1. Active faults:

In home care, patient care is mostly provided by a caregiver in which active failures can be identified as lack of knowledge, lack of training, physical problems, cognitive problems. In the case of a nursing assistant who administers medication, active failures can be found to be related to tasks done quickly, low technical level, lack of adherence to institutional norms (protocols); problems of attention and communication.

2. As contributory factors:

• Inherent to the patient: polymedicated patient, organic mental disorder, uncooperative patient, extreme ages of life, patient with associated morbidities.

• Task-inherent: medication scheduling error, administration error, lack of training, lack of caregiver training, failure to manage clinical records.

• Inherent to technology: failures in the technical use of medicines, shortages, expiration of dates, not having unidosis, not having protocols for dilutions and mixtures.

• Inherent to the team: failures in communication with the patient, carer or other members of the team, failures in supervision, not having the participation and supervision of a pharmaceutical chemist to verify the pharmacotherapeutic profile (mainly in chronic, polymedicated patients and with over-added pathologies or therapeutic failure under study).

• Inherent to the environment: pollution, distractions, home unsuitable for hospitalisation or home care.

• Inherent to the individual (other professionals, family members), communication failures, planning failures, lack of knowledge, lack of training, poor interpersonal relationships.

3. Latent faults: we can find:

• Lack of specific guidelines for home-based care

• No induction, no training within the programme

• Non-authorisation of supplies or medicines

• Route scheduling failures

Safe practices for the prevention of adverse drug reactions in home-based care

1. Barriers to active failures:

• Definition of profiles and competencies, essential requirements to become a carer.

• Training of caregivers

• Specific training, induction and re-induction course for home-based equipment.

• Exclusive training in the management of high-risk medications, drug interactions and adverse drug reactions.

2. The barrier to intervention for non-adherence to standards involves mandatory institutional guidelines, checklist-type controls, monitoring and evaluation.

3. Barriers to contributory factors:

•   Patient: characterisation and identification of risk for each patient

•   Of the task: implementation of checklist-type controls, identification of correct, shift handovers, protocol evaluations, security rounds.

•   For technology: prior verification of drug availability, training on the correct use of high-risk drugs, drug interactions, side effects, dilutions and administration techniques.

•   For the team: effective communication and teamwork techniques, regular supervision.

•   In the environment: minimum criteria for periodical and mandatory home care verification, controlling pollution and distractions, waste management protocol.

•   In individuals: training, induction, re-induction, assertive communication techniques, planning and teamwork.

4. Barriers to latent failures:

The service provider must guarantee supervision activities, expected guidelines for home care, supplies, medicines, equipment maintenance, real time communication with institutional technical support and optimise the scheduling of routes.

11. Phlebitis (chemical or infectious)

For the period analysed, phlebitis was prioritised as the second cause of adverse events, whether of a chemical or infectious cause.

General objective

Minimise risks and possible injuries caused by phlebitis in patients in home care by generating strategies that ensure the correct administration of medicines with the least risk and the best results.

Specific objectives

•   To identify the active failures that exist during the process of administering medicines in home care.

•   Identify contributory factors inherent to the patient, the task and technology, the health care team and the patient's care environment.

•   To define the main latent faults that occur during the administration of medicines that could favour the presence of phlebitis, mainly due to chemical or mechanical causes.

- Establish safety barriers to prevent the occurrence of active failures, contributory factors or latent failures that may favour the occurrence of phlebitis in home care patients.

Outreach

This package applies to the care of patients at home, under the care of a health institution, through a home care team.

Applying the problem-based approach model, under the London protocol model, we have:

1. Active faults:

If an untrained caregiver is involved in the administration of parenteral medicines or is a member of the health care team with a lack of knowledge of protocols, lack of experience, low technical level, physical problems, illness or functional incapacity to perform the task or carry out the activities of care. Conscious non-adherence to institutional norms and protocols.

2. Contributory factors:
- Inherent to the patient: uncooperative, with associated morbidity, skin problems, lack of patient hygiene, patient with behavioural or consciousness problems.
- Task-inherent: lack of institutional protocols, lack of training, lack of supervision, prescription errors, administration errors, errors in aseptic technique and venipuncture.
- Technology-inherent: catheter failures, problems related to dilutions, speed of drug administration, concentrations and mixtures, non-availability of devices or drugs.
- Inherent to the team: communication problems, lack of teamwork, lack of technical support and supervision.
- Inherent to the environment: pollution; overcrowding
- Inherent to the individual: lack of information to patients and relatives, failures in communication with patients and relatives, lack of training, lack of compliance with standards and protocols.

3. Latent failures:

Lack of auditing, supervision, protocols, expected guidelines, lack of induction, re-induction or training, unavailability of supplies, lack of staff knowledge assessment.

Suggested safe practices for the prevention and management of phlebitis:

1. Barriers for active faults:

With the caregiver to have adequate information and communication to help prevent phlebitis; with the treating professional (nurse) training in venipuncture techniques, aseptic technique, management of high-risk medications, drug reactions and interactions, dilutions, mixtures and administration of parenteral medications.

In relation to non-adherence to standards, defined protocols, mandatory guidelines and monitoring

2. Barriers to contributory factors:

•   On the patient: Identifying and prioritising patient risks

•   Task-related: induction, re-induction, training of health personnel (nurses), regular supervision and technical support.

•   In relation to technology: preventing stock-outs of supplies and medicines and training in their correct use

•   In relation to the team: assertive communication techniques with the health team, shift handovers, checklists, cross-checking, safety rounds.

•   In relation to the environment: require and periodically verify minimum safe environmental conditions for a patient receiving parenteral treatment (hand washing, utilities, waste collection and management, safe storage and handling of drugs and devices).

•   In relation to individuals: training in protocols, guidelines for the whole health care team, information and education for patients and carers.

3. Barriers to latent failures:

Regular and effective supervision, prevention of stock-outs of medicines and supplies, induction, re-induction and re-training of the entire health team, timely authorisation of supplies and procedures.

111.   Adverse events secondary to surgery and other procedures

Events related to surgery (post-operative) and other home management procedures have been prioritised as the third cause of adverse events for the period analysed.

General objective

Minimise risks and possible injuries secondary to post-operative or home care procedures, generating strategies that ensure the correct integral care of these patients with the least risk and the best results for the patient and their family.

Specific objectives

• Identify active failures during postoperative or procedural management in home care.

• Identify contributory factors inherent to the patient, the task and technology, the health care team and the patient's care environment.

• Define the main latent failures that occur during postoperative or procedural management that can be managed in home care.

• Establish safety barriers to prevent the occurrence of active failures, contributory factors or latent failures that may favour the occurrence of events secondary to postoperative or procedural management in home care.

Outreach

This package applies to the care of home patients, where postoperative management or procedures are performed during home care under the care of a health care institution, through a care team.

Applying the problem-based approach model, under the London protocol model, we have:

1. Active faults:

If an untrained caregiver participates in the care of the patient or is a member of the health care team with a lack of knowledge of protocols, lack of experience, low technical level, physical problems, illness or functional incapacity to work or perform the activities of care. Conscious non-adherence to institutional norms and protocols.

2. Contributory factors:

• Inherent to the patient: uncooperative, with associated morbidity, skin problems, lack of patient hygiene, overweight patient, patient with alterations in behaviour or consciousness (agitated, in coma, etc.).

• Inherent to the task: lack of institutional protocols, lack of training in device handling (catheters, catheters), lack of training in wound management, dressings, ostomies, lack of supervision, prescription errors, errors in dressing management technique and errors in aseptic technique.

• Inherent to technology: device failures (catheters, syringes), lack of knowledge in handling devices, healing elements and use of technologies.

• Inherent to the team: communication problems, lack of teamwork, lack of technical support and supervision.

- Inherent to the environment: pollution; overcrowding, self-care failures

- Inherent to the individual: lack of information to patients and relatives, failures in communication and training to patients, caregivers and relatives, lack of training, lack of compliance with norms and protocols of the health team.

3. Latent failures:

Lack of auditing, supervision, protocols, expected guidelines, lack of induction, re-induction or training, unavailability of supplies, lack of assessment of staff knowledge, lack of monitoring techniques for devices and their handling.

Suggested safe practices for postoperative and procedural management in home care.

Only those post-operative and procedures that the physician orders to be managed at home should be handled.

1. Barriers for active faults:

With the caregiver to have adequate information and communication to help prevent complications; with the treating professional (nurse) training in wound management techniques, healing, ostomies, catheters, aseptic technique, among others.

In relation to non-adherence to standards, defined protocols, mandatory guidelines (checklist, daily monitoring) and mandatory supervision.

2. Barriers to contributory factors:

- In the patient: Assessment and identification prior to home management of the patient's risks and pre-planning.

- Task-related: induction, re-induction, training of health care personnel (nurses), in aseptic technique, wound management, wound care, dressing, catheters, catheters, ostomies, including regular supervision and technical support by the supervisor and monitoring of the patient and with the help of the caregiver.

- In relation to technology: preventing shortages of supplies and medicines and training in their correct use.

- In relation to the team: assertive communication techniques with the health team, shift handovers, checklists, cross-checking, safety rounds. Permanent communication with patient and caregiver in order to prevent events and warn of risk signs.

- In relation to the environment: require and periodically verify minimum safe environmental conditions for a patient receiving care for wounds, dressings, probes, etc. at home (hand washing, utilities, waste collection and management, safe storage and handling of drugs and devices).

• In relation to individuals: training in protocols, guidelines for the whole health care team, information and education for patients and carers.

3. Barriers to latent failures:

Regular and effective supervision, prevention of stock-outs of medicines and supplies, induction, re-induction and re-training of the entire health team, timely authorisation of supplies and procedures.

IV. Adverse events pressure ulcers.

The fourth leading cause of adverse events for the period analysed was pressure ulcers.

General objective

Minimise risks and possible skin lesions, typical of pressure ulcers.

Specific objectives

• To identify active failures in the management of patients with risk factors for pressure ulcers in home care.
• Identify contributory factors inherent to the patient, the task and technology, the health care team and the patient's care environment related to pressure ulcers.

• To define the main latent failures that occur during the management of patients in home care, which contribute to the occurrence of pressure ulcers.
• Establish safety barriers to prevent the occurrence of active failures, contributory factors or latent failures that may favour the occurrence of pressure ulcers in home care.

Outreach

This package applies to the care of home patients with risk factors for pressure ulcers during their home care, who are under the care of a health care institution, through a home care team.

Applying the problem-based approach model, under the London protocol model, we have:

Active faults:

If an untrained caregiver participates in the care of the patient, he or she will fail due to lack of knowledge, health limitations, age limitations, mobility limitations or competence limitations.

If it is a member of the health team with a lack of knowledge of protocols, lack of experience, low technical level, physical problems, illness or functional incapacity to work or carry out the activities involved. Conscious non-adherence to institutional norms and protocols.

2. Contributory factors:

• Inherent to the patient: uncooperative, with limited morbidity, skin problems, lack of patient hygiene, overweight patient, patient with alterations in behaviour or consciousness (agitated, in coma, uncooperative, etc.).

• Task-inherent: lack of training or protocols for handling skin and mobility-limited patients, patients with prostheses, orthoses or disabilities that affect their mobility, lack of training in wound management, dressings, ostomies, lack of supervision, errors in dressing management techniques and errors in aseptic techniques.

• Inherent to technology: failure of devices for the prevention of skin lesions, lack of knowledge in the handling of devices, failures in the use of healing elements and protection of the skin in areas of pressure.

• Inherent to equipment: communication problems, lack of teamwork, lack of technical support and supervision.

• Inherent to the environment: pollution; overcrowding, self-care failures; overheating and over-breathing.

• Inherent to the individual: lack of information to patients and relatives, failures in communication and training to patients, caregivers and relatives, lack of training, lack of compliance with standards and protocols for position changes and skin management.

3. Latent failures:

Lack of auditing, supervision, protocols, expected guidelines, lack of induction, re-induction or training, unavailability of supplies, lack of assessment of staff knowledge, lack of monitoring techniques for devices and their handling.

Suggested safe practices for prevention and management of skin injuries.

Only skin lesions that the physician authorises home management should be managed at home.

1. Barriers for active faults:

With the caregiver to have adequate information and communication to avoid complications and adverse events; with the treating professional (nurse) training in skin management techniques, changes of position and wound management, cures, ostomies, catheters, aseptic technique, among others.
In relation to non-adherence to standards, defined protocols, mandatory guidelines (checklist, daily monitoring) and mandatory supervision.

2. Barriers to contributory factors:

•   On the patient: Pre-assessment and pre-identification of skin lesion risks for all home management patients and pre-planning.

•   In relation to the task: induction, re-induction, training of health personnel (nurses) in aseptic technique, skin management, timetable changes, wound management and healing, catheters, catheters, ostomies, including regular supervision and technical support by the supervisor and monitoring of the patient and with the help of the caregiver.

•   In relation to technology: preventing shortages of supplies and medicines and training in their correct use.

•   In relation to the team: assertive communication techniques with the health team, shift handovers, checklists, cross-checking, safety rounds. Ongoing communication with patient and caregiver to prevent events and warn of risk signs.

•   In relation to the environment: require and verify on a regular basis minimum conditions of a safe environment for a bedridden patient receiving care at home (minimum facilities: hand washing, utilities, waste collection and management, safe storage and handling of drugs and devices).

•   In relation to individuals: training in protocols, guidelines for the whole health care team, information and education for patients and carers.

3. Barriers to latent failures:
Regular and effective supervision, prevention of stock-outs of medicines and supplies, induction, re-induction and re-training of the entire health team, timely authorisation of supplies and procedures.

Annex B. Proposal of guidelines to build a public policy on safe practices in low complexity home care for the different actors of the system Ministry of Health, territorial entities, system administrators, patients and caregivers.

For the construction of this Public Policy proposal we used the "Diseno de PoPticas Publicas de Franco Corzo, published in July. 2013. Mexico. IEXE editorial" (35)ask

The problem:

Home care, when carried out in an environment adapted for housing and not for providing medical care, makes the provision of health services more risky, facilitating the occurrence of adverse events that can even lead to the death of the patient; being these events mostly preventable, through the implementation of safe care practices, could their effects be prevented or mitigated?

Importance of the problem

Adverse events and incidents in home care occur with an incidence of 6.8% and a prevalence of 11.2% (APEAS study), in home care services throughout the world, with a very significant under-reporting in Colombia where in the population analysed they occur with a prevalence of 1.0% with social and functional costs for patients and their families, which can range from the death of a patient, sequelae, additional costs for the additional management required by these adverse events.

Multi-causal analysis of the problem

In identifying the causes that lead to the need for public policy, we find the following:

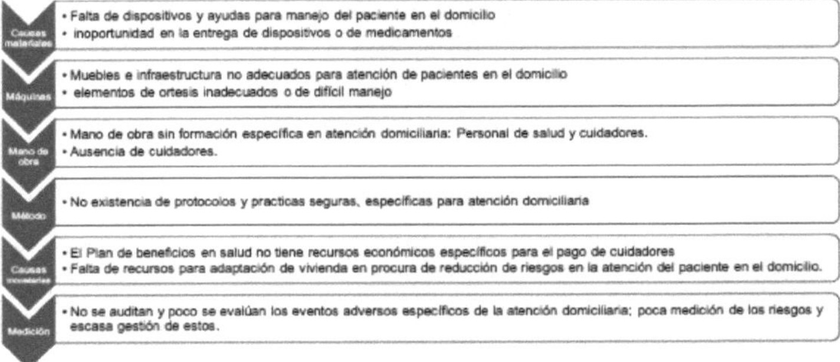

Prioritised adverse events in home care.

Of the events identified in the sample studied and the Pareto methodology applied, the following correspond to 77% of the events identified:

1- Adverse drug reaction with 31%.

2- Phlebitis with 18%.

3- Events related to surgeries or some procedures with 15%.

4- Pressure ulcers with 13%.

Safety practices in home care today:

5- Train the health care team in safe home care practices that are ideally adapted to the home.

6- Training of some caregivers on more necessary topics for the patient.

7- Patient, family and caregiver education

8- Family caregivers who adapt the home and learn from daily practice.

Suggested best practices:

9- Home-based care training packages.

10- Specific training in risk management in home care for the health care team; carers, patients and relatives.

11- The need for a specific profile for a home care carer: technical and non-technical.

12- The need for specific criteria for home care.

13- Need to include the caregiver in the POS.

14- Importance of promoting home care safety in the patient safety programme.

15- Implementation of risk management in patient safety in home care.

Costs incorporating security in home-based care.

National level (Ministry of Health and Social Protection):

16- Include safe home care practices in the national patient safety programme.

17- Take home-based care into account in the criteria to be developed in health habilitation.

18- Define a percentage of the health benefit plan to support the costs of home care (Percentage of P&P in the home patient).

19- Include in the staff requirements the profile of carers: technical and non-technical.

At the regional level (Departmental and District Health Secretariats):

Comply with the verification of defined minimum requirements (Habilitacion) in home care programmes.

20- Include in Surveillance and Control, the verification of patient safety at home.

For Administrators

21- Definition of a percentage of the UPC (Unidad de pago por capitacion) for home care (caregiver, care aids, devices, medicines at home, transport if necessary, procedures at home).

22- Patient safety policy and programme, including home-based care.

23- Audit and control of the technical management of home care.

24- Increased promotion of home-based care.

For providers

25- Patient safety policy and programme, including home-based care.

26- Audit and control of the technical management of home care.

27- Increased promotion of home-based care.

28- Training of specific health team in home care (safe practices in home care).

For carers, patients and relatives

29- Specific conditions in the home, to ensure safety in home care.

30- Specific training for home care.

31- Knowledge of safe practices and risk management in home care.

Nowadays, EPS and IPS offer home care to a greater number of users in hospitalisation at home; chronic patients, palliative care patients and older adults, among others. A worldwide prevalence of 11.2% adverse events in home care has been identified; in the study population of 1002 patients in home care, 40 adverse events were identified, with an incidence of 3.9% in the IPS related to the study.

Annex C. Interview with patients, relatives and carers

Date: City:

The objective:

This interview is part of an academic work where we want to know about your experiences as patients, relatives or caregivers during home care on issues related to safety in CARE.

Given the current pandemic situation, this targeted interview will be conducted by telephone by the investigators and will not be recorded.

This interview is completely voluntary and if you do not agree to participate in it at any time you may indicate this and withdraw and it will in no way affect your normal care process that you receive from the health institution.

Important concepts:

0 **Good safety practices**: "Technical recommendations that are voluntarily applied by health care personnel, the patient and the caregiver during the home care process to prevent, control or reduce the risk of injury or harm to the patient".

0 **Home care (WHO),** is the care provided at the patient's home, including comprehensive health care.

Respected patients, family members and caregivers, this telephone interview has a few questions that the researcher will ask you to answer briefly, but honestly, according to what you experience during your home care process.

QUESTIONS:

32- Have the professionals providing your home care given you explanations about safe practices during care?

Yes: __ No: ___ Yes: __ No: ___ Yes: __ No: ___ Yes: __ No: ___

33- If your answer above is YES, please indicate which explanations you have been given, most frequently, please choose one option:

POSSIBLE RESPONSE	YES
What are safe practices:	
On risks during home care	
Prevention of injury or damage	
Other, which one:	

34- Do you remember if at any time during your treatment at home, did any of your caregivers explain to you how to prevent any type of risk from your home care, please choose one option?

RESPONSE	YES
Risk of falls	
Risk of infection	
Risk of harm from medicines	
Other, which one:	
Risks have never been explained to me	

35- How do you remember most frequently being told about risks that may occur during home care?

RESPONSE	YES
I have been given a primer (Written material)	
I have been explained with images (Rota folio, video).	
I am left with tasks to put into practice	
Verbal explanation only	
Other, which one:	

36- What would you suggest to take into account to improve the explanation given by

the health care team to patients, relatives and caregivers on how to prevent risks
related to care? care   home care?

37- What risks do you identify that you may face during home care by any of the
home-based health care team, choose only one answer:

RESPONSE	YES
Risk of falls	
Risk of infection	
Drug risk	
Risks of skin ulcers	
Risk with serum placement	
Other, which one:	

38- Do you think that the recommendations given to you by health professionals in
HOME CARE need to be improved? Choose only one answer.

RESPONSE	YES
The explanation	
Time spent explaining	
Giving something in writing	
Other, which one:	

39- Do you believe that the risks of injury or harm that occur to patients during home
care are the responsibility of (Choose only one answer)

RESPONSE	YES
Exclusively from the health professional	
Of the patient and the caregiver	
From the EPS	
Of all	

40- How do you or your caregiver experience these good practices during HOME
CARE, how have they helped you, please choose one answer?

RESPONSE	YES
Just listen to them	
I listen and learn	
I put them into practice	
With what we learn we have avoided problems	

41- For the risks you have experienced during home care, which good practices do you consider most important, prioritise one answer?

RESPONSE	YES
Careful with medicines	
Careful with diet	
Caution with cures	
How to avoid falls	
Other, which one:	

42- How does the health care team, as a patient or caregiver, teach you about GOOD SAFETY PRACTICE in HOME CARE; prioritise a response?

RESPONSE	YES
He gives me examples	
Practises with the patient	
They only explain to me verbally	
Video, booklet or flyer	
Other, which one:	

43- What do you propose to improve the home-based care programme, to be considered as GOOD CARE PRACTICE, prioritise one answer?

RESPONSE	YES
More staff available	
Less red tape	
Further explanations	
More services at home, which ones:	

Other, which one:	

44- In your experience, what do you consider to be most at risk during your home care, rate the most at risk with 5, the least with 4, 3 or 2 and the lowest risk with 1, in the items below:

a- Medicines:

b- Professionals: __

c- Administrative procedures:

d- Medical equipment used: __

e- Inappropriate house facilities: ___

f- Other, which:

Annex D. Survey of health system leaders

Objective: Respected professional, this survey is part of an academic research project, which aims to learn about existing guidelines for safe home care practices in health care institutions in Colombia.

I understand that this survey is for academic purposes and I authorise the use of the information provided here for that purpose. I am aware that this is a risk-free investigation and has the approval of the research committee of the institution where the study is being carried out and of the Fundacion Universitaria Juan N. Corpas.

Date: City: Position:

Entity where the respondent works:

Respondent's profession: Gender:

The information from these surveys will be used only for academic purposes for this research and will be stored in the researchers' file in PDF format and tabulated in Excel.

Basic concepts

0 **Good safety practices:** "Technical recommendations of voluntary application by the actors of the Obligatory System of Health Care Quality Assurance of the General System of Social Security in Health" (Technical guideline of good patient safety practices, sectorial unit of standardisation, Ministry of Social Protection).

0 **Home care (WHO)** is a form of programmed care that brings biopsychosocial and spiritual care and attention to the patient's home.

Questions with only one answer:

45- What guidelines do you know about good safety practices in home care in our country?

46- What guidelines on safe practice in home care are available to the organisation you represent?

47- How these guidelines in practice contribute to improving safety in home-based care:

48- What adjustments do you recommend to promote improvements in good safety practices in home care today?

49- What are the risks in home care that justify good safe care practices?

50- What evidence exists in the organisation you represent of measurement of safe practices and risks identified in home care?

51- Can this evidence be shared for this research?

IF: __

NO: __

52- How do you think patients and families can be involved in the development of these good safety practices?

53- How does your institution assess the degree of understanding of patients and caregivers of these safety practices in home care?

54- What difficulties for the application of safe practices in home care do you identify from the organisation you represent?

55- How good practice guidelines are adapted and applied to home-based care.

56- Are these safe practices specifically adapted for home-based care?

Yes: NO: ___

Why:

13- What positive indicators of safe practice in home care have been identified, can the available evidence be shared?

14. Has the institution you represent learned anything from the implementation or evaluation of safe home care practices?

YES: ___ NO:

Because:

15- Is the topic of safe practices in home care included in your organisation's training plan?

YES: ___ NO: ___

Because:

16- How has this training in "Good practice in home care" been reflected in your care process?

17- When implementing safe home care practices, which impact outcomes do you find most relevant? (Please rank in order of priority from 1 to 5, with 5 being the most important to you and 1 being the least important on the list):

The prevention of injuries to the patient:

The prevention of consequences for the family:

Avoid cost overruns in the care process:

To maintain the patient's confidence in the institution:

Avoid lawsuits:

Other, which one:

18- In implementing safe home care practices, have you been able to identify the concept of patient and family experience?

YES: ___ NO: ___

Because:

Annex E. Survey of home care professionals

Objective: Respected professional, this survey is part of an academic research project that aims to know guidelines for safe practices in home care in health institutions in Colombia. The completion of this survey is purely voluntary.

I understand that this survey is for academic purposes and I therefore authorise the use of the information provided here for this purpose. I am aware that there is no major risk in the handling of this information, as it has the endorsement of the institution where the study is being carried out and the researchers will provide us with institutional feedback.

Date: City: Position:

Respondent's profession: Gender:

Additional training in:

Years of experience in home care work: years.

Basic concepts

0 **Good safety practices**: "Technical recommendations of voluntary application by the actors of the Obligatory System of Quality Assurance of Health Care of the General System of Social Security in Health" (Technical guideline of good patient safety practices, sectorial unit of standardisation, Ministry of Social Protection).
0 **Home care** (WHO) is a form of programmed care that brings biopsychosocial and spiritual care and attention to the patient's home.

For questions 1 to 12, please prioritise your answer and indicate the option you consider to be the most important.

26- Are you aware of guidelines on good patient safety practices in home care? YES NO

27- If you answered **YES to** the previous question, where do you know them from, please indicate the possible answer:

POSSIBLE RESPONSE	YES
Guidelines given by the IPS where he/she works	
Guidelines given by a different institution	

28- If you have received extra-institutional guidelines for safe practice in home care, you have acquired these guidelines from:

POSSIBLE RESPONSE	Only one
International guidelines	
National Guidelines	
Undergraduate training only	
Another training, which one:	

29- In the organisation where you work, training in good safe practices in home care is promoted: YES   NO

5- If in the previous question (question 3) you answered **YES** training is promoted where you work, how is it promoted?

POSSIBLE RESPONSE	Only one
It is trained by the same institution	
Subsidizes training at an educational institution	
It only gives you permission to study	
Other, which one:	

6- If you receive training in safe practices where you work in home care, this training is:

POSSIBLE RESPONSE	Only one

Specifies in Good safety practice in home-based care	
In security training, but **not specific** to home care.	
Event and incident reporting only	
Other, which one:	

7- In the institution where you work, how do you inform patients and carers about safe practices in HOME CARE?

POSSIBLE RESPONSE	Only one
It is demonstrated with examples	
They are given lectures on safe practices.	
Patients and carers are left with tasks	
Other, which one:	
They are not informed	

8- In the institution where you work, what are the main risks in home care?

POSSIBLE RESPONSE	YES
Risks related to medicinal products	
Risks related to infections	
Related to the ca^das	
Related to skin care	
Another risk, which:	

9- In the institution where you work as a home care professional, how do you do the impact assessment of good safety practices in home care?

POSSIBLE RESPONSE	YES
By means of security indicators in Home Care	
Qualifying what patients and carers have learnt	
Assessing practitioners' knowledge	
Assessing events and incidents.	

Other, which one:	

10- In the implementation of good security practices in HOME CARE, prioritise one option that you would suggest to make them more effective:

POSSIBLE RESPONSE	Only one
Safe practices exclusive to home-based care	
Include them in the training plan.	
To give us more elements to work with	
Frequent evaluation	
Other method, which one:	

11- Do you know the main impact that the implementation of good safety practices in home-based care has had in your institution?

POSSIBLE RESPONSE	YES
It has had no impact	
Fewer patient injuries	
Impact on costs	
Impact on the qualification of professionals	
Another impact, which:	

12- Since its work at home, it has prioritised which adverse events have been improved through the implementation of good safety practices in home care.

POSSIBLE RESPONSE	YES
No improvement of adverse events has been achieved.	
Infection-related events have been improved	
Risks related to falls have been improved	
Skin care related events have been improved.	
Another event, which:	

13- Do you know if the institution where you work has a manual or instructions on good security practices in HOME CARE?

POSSIBLE RESPONSE	YES
There is a manual or instruction manual on good practice in home care.	
Just some good practices, but **not specific for home care**	
Other practices, which ones:	

Multiple choice questions, for grading and prioritisation.

14- If you could include in the training plan where you work, training in good security practices in HOME CARE, please rate in order of importance the following: (PRIORITIZE your answers from 1 to 5, with 1 being the least important to 5 being the most important, please number each one accordingly):

a- What are good safety practices in home care and how do professionals implement them?

b- Protocol for reporting adverse events in HOME CARE...:

c- Inform patients and caregivers how to implement good home care safety practices:

__ __ __ c- Inform patients and caregivers how to implement good home care safety practices: __

d- Protocol for the analysis and improvement of adverse events in HOME CARE: __

e- How to assess the correct implementation of good practices in HOME CARE: __

15- From your professional experience, do you consider that the implementation of good safety practices in home care **can contribute to** (Please rate and prioritise your answers, ask from 1 to 5, with 1 being the least important, in your opinion, and 5 being the most important):

a- Avoid harm to the patient:

b- Avoid lawsuits:

c- Maintain the confidence of the patient and his or her family: __

d- Improve reputation: __

e- Prevent cost overruns:

f- Other, which:

Annex F. Informed consent for interviewing patients, family members and caregivers of the home care programme

Respected patients and caregivers, this interview that we want to do with you, is part of a research project that is being carried out as a degree project in the Master of Public Health at the Fundacion Universitaria Juan N. Corpas in the city of Bogota.

The purpose of this survey is to identify experiences you have had during your home care. The purpose of this survey is purely academic and its completion is voluntary, and each of you may withdraw from the interview when you consider it appropriate, without affecting the normal provision of your health services.

This research does not generate risk because it is limited to a retrospective analysis of the experiences and knowledge of the patients, relatives and caregivers interviewed, and it preserves the confidentiality of the persons interviewed by recording the initial letters of their full name and their identification number.

Knowing clearly the purpose of the present interview, I authorise the use of the information I am able to give here, for eminently academic purposes.

I fill out the survey voluntarily, knowing before filling it out that my name will not appear in the survey, nor that of my caregiver, I authorize the professionals in charge of the study: Lida Beltran and Yesid Ram^ez, the use of this information, as part of the academic research that they are carrying out in the Master of Public Health.

Given in Bogota on this day of   the month of   of 2021

Patient's signature:

Caregiver signature:

Initials of first names and surnames:

Initials of name:

Document no:

Document No:

Respected patient, relative or caregiver, if you require related information, we

offer you a contact telephone number:

<u>**Dissent**</u>

I   ,   at   date

I do not authorize Dr. Lida Beltran and Dr. Yesid Ram^ez, Master of Public Health students, to include me in this interview as part of an academic research **proposal on safe practices and procedures for low complexity home care.**

I therefore sign:

Patient's signature:

Caregiver signature:

Initials of first names and surnames:

Initials of name:

Document no:

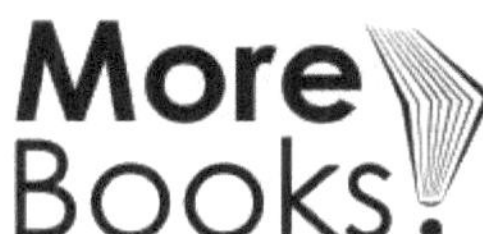
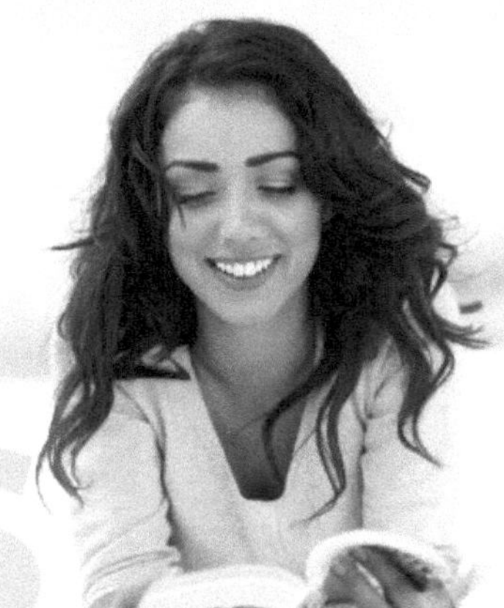

I want morebooks!

Buy your books fast and straightforward online - at one of world's fastest growing online book stores! Environmentally sound due to Print-on-Demand technologies.

Buy your books online at
www.morebooks.shop

Kaufen Sie Ihre Bücher schnell und unkompliziert online – auf einer der am schnellsten wachsenden Buchhandelsplattformen weltweit! Dank Print-On-Demand umwelt- und ressourcenschonend produziert.

Bücher schneller online kaufen
www.morebooks.shop

info@omniscriptum.com
www.omniscriptum.com

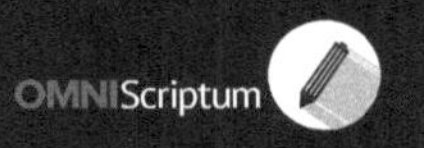

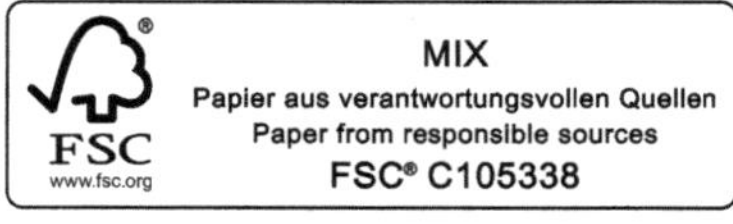

Printed by Books on Demand GmbH, Norderstedt / Germany